# Living Well
# with Lyme

*Also by Caroline Sojourner*

# Total Healing
# to the Limits of Living

A Sourcebook for Awakening and Engaging
the Healing Energies
of the Tree of Life

# Living Well With Lyme

## A Handbook for Self-Healers of Lyme, Chronic Fatigue, and Fibromyalgia

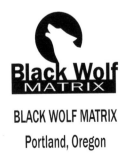

BLACK WOLF MATRIX

Portland, Oregon

ISBN 978-0-9667743-5-1
Printed in the United States of America in 2015

Black Wolf Matrix
Portland, OR
www.livinghighwithlyme.com

# Testimonials to Information Posted on My Blog

After putting some of the information in this book out on my *livinghighwithlyme* blog I received these testimonials about the effectiveness of natural healing. Posts have not been edited except for names.

Hello Caroline, I have Dercum's Disease (DD or Adiposa Dolorosa AD) and was very close to despair with myriad symptoms and complications of this unfortunate and very rare condition. DD can present as Lyme disease and this is how I came to find your elegant paper; the info therein has been a lifesaver.

I've been taking Glutathione (reduced) for the past few months. Already my tumours have reduced in size by 50%. The attendant 'brain fog' and the eczematous rash in my ears (which many doctors denied could occur) have almost disappeared. I want to shout it from the rooftops: Allelulia for Glutathione & Caroline.

It's still early days but I hope Glutathione continues to astound me by reducing my pain, among other things. THANK YOU, SO MUCH, for your informative, highly readable yet academic blog. J

*A later post from this reader:*

I'm still taking Glutathione (reduced) and it really has helped me enormously but I've added quercetin, serrapeptase and beta-glucans *inter alia*. The new additions are working their magic too. I am more energised and because the tumours around my torso have reduced somewhat, I can now bend down & get up more easily. The pain is more manageable too. Hurrah. Jude.

Dear Caroline, I am part of a clinical research project on glutathione. We will be presenting our findings at the Fascia Research Congress in March 2012. Your explanation of methylation and your Celtic knot graphic are superb and I would like your permission to borrow them to use in our presentation. K. S.

What a well-written article! Thank you for the information. I do have methylation cycle pathway block, Lyme and a whole host of co-infections and viruses, other infections. I have been taking substances to help with this block, as well as glutathione IVs, and am aware of many facts, but this article cleared up some questions and described more than what I had been able to find elsewhere. Again, thank you so much! I also do EWOT at home and it helps me with my energy levels and overall feeling better when I do it regularly. P. K.

I've been using ozone for 8 months for Lyme. Before I started I couldn't work even from home and barely could leave the house. In the past 8 months I've been able to move out of my mom's house and secure a good job and start working 3/4 time. Ozone has been the most effective thing I've used for getting my life back, and I have used long-term antibiotics, Bicillin shots, herbs, etc. Something about the oxygenation and detox really helps for getting back on track. A. R.

I found this information to be very well written. I have Auto-Immune Dysfunction & am trying to heal myself with Ozone & a nutritional therapy called the Gerson therapy. People heal from every kind of disease such as cancer, diabetes, aids, Lyme, etc. Just on the therapy alone, the Ozone adds wellness, which helps an individual deal with the day to day challenges of living with a disease . . . I first bought the equipment & tried to heal myself with it alone, but I was missing the nutritional piece, once I found that with Gerson, then I was missing the feeling of wellness while doing the therapy, as it is an arduous therapy that can take as long as 3 years to cure a disease, such as cancer or Lyme, which per Charlotte Gerson, is harder to cure than Cancer. People have cured cancer by going on a raw food diet for 10 months alone. That being said the same could apply for Lyme. Ultimately, the only thing that is going to heal a person is their own "Immune, Hormone, Enzyme, Mineral & Organ Systems." Nutrition in & garbage out, this is the only way to truly heal a body. We are all oxygen deprived due to wrong diets, polluted air, food, water & all the anaerobic microbes that use our bodies, as their homes. The amazing thing about the human body is that it is very resilient & will keep trying till the very last moment, as long as the spirit does not give up hope. Faith & Love Heals All! God Bless – SAL

Just stumbled across your site. What a thoughtful and well written insight on attitude and healing. I am something of a medical renegade myself in dealing with chronic Lyme and all the debilitating accompanying nasties. Most enjoyed and share your point of view. To your grand health, Cathy

Dear Caroline... what a magnificent spirit you have. I've dealt with auto immune problems myself, having severe arthritis in my 20s and told at the time I would never walk again. It took years. I still have moments when I forget to be 'disciplined' as you said, although I do allow myself to have something foolish now and then. You're right about the antibiotics! All best, Sam

Excellent, clearly presented information!!! Absolutely indispensible for anyone wanting to improve their health. I would add that Earthing to replenish one's store of electrons and mitigate the effects of EMF can also make a big difference in how one feels, how fast one heals, and in one's energy levels. (see "Earthing: the most important health discovery ever?" by Clinton Ober et al., visit http://www.earthinginstitute.net/ or listen to Dr Joseph Mercola's interview with Clinton Ober on YouTube). Thank you very much for making this info available. B. D.

**Dedicated to all who choose to heal with nature.**

*To change one's life: start immediately.*
*Do it flamboyantly.*
*No exceptions.*

William James

# Contents

# Preface

## Why I Am Writing This Book

*In order to arrive at a place you do not know,*
*you must go by a way you do not know.*

St. John of the Cross

*I do not wish to hear about the moon*
*from someone who has not been there.*

Mark Twain.

The most useful information on disease has come from
those people who have been diagnosed with a condition
and can articulate how they have mastered it or learned
to live a fulfilling life in spite of it. We ask them especially about the details of the actual healing: what it felt
like and what sensations, thoughts or behaviors accompanied or preceded the healing process.

Jean Achterberg

Lyme can be a source of prolonged, relentless suffering, particularly in the early years. In seeking relief from this I usually found that
answers too easily gained were somewhat of a disappointment and
a letdown—I like the struggle. But this struggle with Lyme has
been about as close to my existential limits as I would ever want to
venture. For the first ten years I felt like I was being tortured from
within my own skull; my central nervous system felt naked and

disrobed. I began to realize that this strange territory of suffering was an intensive challenge in personal growth.

One day I opened a book by Claude Steiner to these words which described what I had been experiencing for the previous ten years:

> Going crazy is an utterly terrifying experience in which nighttime is filled with sleeplessness or nightmares and infinite fear and dread, and in which daytime is fraught with incapacity to act, unwillingness to move, contempt and abuse from others, confusion, disorganization, suspicion, despair, and a recurring wish to end one's life and be done with it.

Somehow the voice of hope kept company with me, even in the worst times. I knew there had to be a way out. It offended my sense of the fitness of things to think it was hopeless. I felt a connection to every person in every age who has ever suffered: this made me feel I was not alone with this. But still there was no place to run to or hide. Every moment was a repeat of the moment before. I was stuck in a movie where the horseman was charging towards me over and over again. Sometimes I could stand up to the challenge without flinching or running and sometimes I could only fall into the black hole of despair.

# An Outlook for Recovering

The underlying disturbances in normal physiological functioning of various organ systems are a set-up for suffering and depression. Therefore, square one in restoring a healthier frame of mind is to address underlying physiological imbalances by whatever means available. In this book I offer some tools that I have found useful for healing. Much of the psychological disruption and social alienation that accompanies illness seems to improve rapidly when the body is restored to healthy function.

When we come, sooner or later, to the realization that allopathic interventions do not really heal Lyme or chronic fatigue, it becomes apparent that the only alternative, if we do not want to stay sick forever, is to launch ourselves whole-heartedly into a program of natural self-healing. We must honor our native desire for wholeness, for wisdom, and for energy. We must learn to become so in touch with our body that we can intuit what we need whenever symptoms take a turn this way or that way or any old way.

Thirty years of dealing with Lyme surprises has led me deeper and deeper into natural healing. I have gradually settled into a personal protocol that is easy to do with regularity. Perhaps if I were a paragon of self-discipline I could heal the disease completely. But I have to work with who I am and what I am capable of doing: I do manage to keep the Lyme under control and remain more or less functional.

It has taken me this long to learn to work within my personal capabilities and still overcome symptoms. I could not have written anything useful twenty years ago or even ten years ago—I had to learn to trust my intuition, my instincts, and my personal research to find the right combination of commitment and doing. When I started out the only option was antibiotics, for the world was just becoming aware of this disease. The only natural therapy anyone knew about was to take lots of vitamin C. Not much happened in the way of healing.

Antibiotics were effective at first, but when they stopped working I realized that it would be pretty difficult to feel any worse. I decided to get off them no matter what. I found instant relief in heat therapies, particularly hot tubs and saunas. The next step was my discovery of ozone and oxygen therapies, my mainstay for many years now. When I started taking B12 shots my "major depression" changed overnight.

After years of Band-Aid answers to symptoms I have pretty much had to fall back on my own intelligence and intuition. No more "maybe this/maybe that" shotgun approach to symptoms. I want to heal my whole being. I will use anything that works for me whether it meets mainstream approval or not. In my research of medical journals I found writers who deny the effectiveness of many alternative therapies. I can only state categorically that except for long-term, expensive (and controversial) intravenous hydrogen peroxide therapy, I have made more cumulative and lasting progress under my own self-determined protocols than I have with office visits and IV drips.

The hardest, and perhaps most vital, lesson to learn was the importance of self-discipline and persistence even when things were going well. Trying to heal oneself sometimes feels like trying to pull yourself out of quicksand: the more you struggle, the more you get pulled back. But with committed effort and the right protocol it can be done. Just doing herbs when you have flare ups, or just doing ozone once in a while is not enough.

You must fundamentally rebuild your body, your immune system, and your way of looking at life. It may look overwhelming, especially if you are in the depleted physical and financial situations in which many subjects find themselves. But the survivor and lover-of-life in us tells us that we have no choice but to engage with it.

# My Ideal Personal Protocol Must Be:

**Doable:** it must be humanly achievable, not requiring heroic levels of self-discipline.

**Effective:** it must show some positive results.

**Affordable:** getting well should not require a big bank account.

**Immune Supportive:** it goes beyond common sense to destroy the immune system with therapies that leave you damaged for life.

**Growth Enhancing:** connecting with our self-healing genius is an opportunity to grow both psychically and spiritually.

# Who Can Benefit From This Book?

This book is for long-term sufferers of Lyme and other mysterious syndromes such as chronic fatigue, fibromyalgia, and many auto-immune disorders. It is for people whose determination to live, no matter what it takes, comes from deep within the self. I believe that if more information were available, more people would take their healing into their own hands. I have attempted to show that total healing consists of finding the pieces that work and linking them into a comprehensive whole.

I offer this book to those who are unhappy with conventional answers and want to want to pursue their own healing but don't know where to start. Self-healing begins, of necessity, with physical healing, leading ultimately to our expansion into wider dimensions of being human.

# Prerequisites for Healing

1. Personal involvement and commitment

2. Doing for yourself

3. Gentleness to self, not overwhelming mind or body

4. Willingness to view healing as an opportunity for inner growth

5. Empowerment and encouragement from self and others

6. Willingness to go beyond the false comforts of conventional wisdom

7. Common sense in knowing when to get help from others (including the medical profession)

# Outline of the Book

This book will suggest a number of approaches to healing:

### 1. Understanding the Challenger and Finding Imagery for Working with the Deeper Mind

Chapter 1, "Spirochete Kingdom Come" offers some preliminary thoughts about the peculiarities, likes, and dislikes of the Lyme spirochete. Understanding this organism is the first step to devising a strategy for outsmarting it.

### 2. Attitude, Determination, and Natural Methods

Chapter 2, "Natural Healing and the Self-Healing Frame of Mind "presents some observations about natural healing and what it might take to be able to practice it.

### 3. The Fundamentals of Immunity

Chapter 3, "Build a Strong Immune System" defines some of the basic terms relating to the immune system. Attention is paid to the TH1/TH2 hypothesis; the role of the intestinal tract (Gut and Physiology Syndrome); and to the function of glutathione and the methylation cycle in supporting immunity. Several methods of restoring immunity are suggested.

### 4. Clearing and Making Room for Healing

Chapter 4, "Good Housekeeping" suggests ways to rid the body of toxins that devastate the nervous system. Methods include neutralizing these toxins through the liver and lymph system. This is easily addressed through simple physical methods and herbs.

### 5. Food as a Healing Ally

Chapter 5, "Plant Power" explores foods that are known to fortify us against disease. Particularly important are the green leafy foods and the high-powered foods such as spirulina, wheatgrass juice, and some common medicinal spices from the kitchen.

Chapter 6, "Ground Zero: What Are You Eating These Days?" lists foods known to exacerbate or even cause symptom flare-ups. Other foods may help to repair the autoimmune response, leaky gut syndrome, and candida. Specific foods help to restore the methylation cycle and minimize nerve symptoms. A Paleo-lithic style diet offers some valuable principles in construct-ing a healing diet: it emphasizes the elimination of man-made foods and incorporation of the foods our bodies are designed to need and digest.

Chapter 7, "Living High with Food" includes a discussion of en-ergy, how it works in the body and how raw foods, juices, and smoothies provide energy. We acknowledge that rigid diets are difficult to maintain, and that dietary changes do take time.

### 6. The Most Effective and Appropriate Supplements

Chapter 8, "A Little Help from Supplements" is a pared-down list of supplements useful for long-term maintenance and res-toration of wellbeing. I personally have mixed feelings about the abundance of supplements being sold these days, but the supplements I have chosen for this list seem to be fairly essen-tial.

### 7. Heat Shock Therapies to Stimulate the Immune Response Known as "Heat Shock"

Chapter 9, "Spirochetes Hate Heat" shows how heat therapies need to be part of any protocol for Lyme because spirochetes cannot live in high heat. Several good ways to incorporate heat into our healing routine are described.

### 8. Increasing Oxygen Intake

Chapter 10, "Cellular Respiration" discusses how insufficient oxygen in the body can reduce the energy needed for basic existence and be a factor in chronic fatigue. Oxygen may be increased through self-administered home ozone treatments and EWOT (exercise with oxygen).

Chapter 11, "Active Breathing" explains what conscious breath work can do to increase energy levels and describes several gentle Ayurvedic breath routines. Other intensive and energetic *pranayama* routines which have been credited with healing Lyme are also described.

### 9. The Deep Mind as the Driver of the Immune System

Chapter 12, "Spirit" introduces tools for holographic healing using the deeper mind. Disease is an entity that responds to metaphor, image, and story. Deeper and slower brain states restore the willingness of the body to counteract stress and its side-effects. Basic methods are suggested: meditation, binaural beat music, loving the self with words and imagery, and simple, meditative breathing. This kind of self-exploration and meditation is easy to learn and has been shown to be a potent tool in creating a mind-set for healing.

### 10. Getting Started

Chapter 13, "A Workable Program" describes what to look for in putting together a natural healing program. Where can we start, and how do we sabotage our healing efforts with the things we do? I reveal the program which seems to work for me. I encourage others to devise their own workable program.

11. **Appendix A:** "Life-Friendly Recipes" is a basic compendium of living foods recipes to incorporate into a healing diet.

12. **Appendix B:** "The Gerson Program" is an overview of a successful program that has been able to heal many serious illnesses.

# Acknowledgments

I would like to acknowledge the naturopathic physicians who try to understand Lyme and other mysterious illnesses: Dr. Satya Ambrose for her loving acupuncture treatments and her belief in me, Dr. Sheryl Deroin for introducing me to ozone, Dr. Mike Conway for valiant struggles with IV needles; and Dr. Jennifer Means for willingness to support me in anything I wanted to try. I am also grateful to my fellow writers and publishers Jean Sheldon and Veronica Esagui for moral support and information sharing. Thank you to Julie Zehetbauer and Marsha Graham for encouraging words. Thanks also to friends and family who believed in this project. Great appreciation and thanks to Rob Abramowitz for allowing me to use his piece on infrared light bulbs. And I send utmost gratitude to Kelly Thompson for his generous and beautiful formatting of this book.

# ONE

# Spirochete Kingdom Come

*When health is absent,*
*wisdom cannot reveal itself;*
*art cannot become manifest;*
*strength cannot be exerted;*
*wealth is useless,*
*and reason is powerless.*

Herophiles, 300 B.C., Father of Anatomy

**Imagery**: I begin this book with a brief look into the power of image, the goal being to encourage each person to collect their own imagery for use in their deeper work. Imagery and metaphor, rather than word, is the language of healing.

## The Challenger

Lyme disease could be understood as a challenge to the human soul to become more sober, to find a way to the essence and real meaning of life. In this way, disease is often a strict taskmaster, a mirror of karma, and it can be a teacher, a guru, for souls who have lost their bearings.

Wolf D. Storl [1]

Illness, especially if it is prolonged, can take us to a threshold beyond which most humans are reluctant to willingly go. Life becomes disrupted and disoriented. A disorienting state of affairs has cornered us and is relentlessly demanding our attention. We become strangers in a strange land. We sense the answers lie within, but for the moment, we cannot find them. There is no escape until and unless we attend to this immediate situation. Illness is a "liminal" experience that threatens to unsettle our very existence unless we make radical changes in how we live. The Lyme presence invades the body so thoroughly and tenaciously that it eats away at us, altering our fundamental physical, mental, and spiritual essence.

## The Spirochete Boogie Woogie

The Lyme organism itself is a metaphor for the disease. Its long, spiral-shaped cells get energy from the oxidation of glucose just like we do. The organism is so constructed that it twists about in a sort of boogie-woogie, changing form to avoid detection. Lyme disease is known for its ability to mimic or induce many neurological conditions, boogying from one symptom to the next.

Bodily and dynamically, spirochetes function like a corkscrew, looking like tightly twisted spiral telephone cords. They are built for destruction: they move by rotating like a drill, boring their way into flesh. Once they have a foothold they drill into our organs, screw up our life, and are very difficult to remove once in place. Anyone contending with long-term Lyme knows that they are up against a pretty "screwy" adversary.

The Lyme adversary may or may not kill directly, but it silently hacks away at our life and vitality. It can kill a lot of what we thought we knew about our self and our life.

**An adversary of this kind demands that we drop everything else to contend with it!**

## Spirochetes Demand Total Attention

They want to invade us emotionally, spiritually, and financially. They want to decide how we are in this world, what emotions we exhibit: they like it best if we are depressed, angry, suicidal, and hopeless. They try to destroy us spiritually, although in time we may come to realize that the fight is actually making us stronger in many ways. They want us to spend all our money on them, and if we don't, too bad for us: they will make life so miserable that we end up buying any old thing we think might help us.

# What do Spirochetes Thrive on?

To outsmart this adversary we need to know what it likes and what it doesn't like. Anything it likes stimulates them to reproduce. We need to explore and adopt life habits that discourage it from having millions of babies.

### 1. Spirochetes Love our Chaos and Stress

Spirochetes prosper on the stress we create through bad habits and unhealthy food and drink. Stress is their maypole party—they congregate and multiply with delight. Stress will damage the immune system and spirochetes love a damaged immune system.

The importance of minimizing stress is well known to Lyme people. A little stress brings on dizziness and possible flare-ups. Symptoms of stress include tiredness, dizziness, confusion, memory problems, irregular heartbeat, difficulty breathing, headaches, muscle tension, low sex drive, nausea, digestive irregularities, depression, fearfulness, restlessness, inability to relax or get proper sleep, and eating too much or too little.

### Sources of Stress

- Too much TV (especially programs that arouse anxiety such as the evening news and gory crime shows)

- Inability to cope with life due to suppressed anger, self-hatred, despair, depression, guilt, negativity, worry, and anxiety

- Dysfunctional relationships that need to be healed or avoided

- Tobacco, alcohol (including alcohol mouthwashes), caffeine, and drugs

- Environmental pollution from chemicals such as formaldehyde (from new carpeting and furniture); household solvents such as paint thinners; pesticides and fungicides; radiation from computers, TVs, electric blankets, heating pads, heated waterbeds, and electric clocks

- Too little or too much exercise

- Inadequate or interrupted sleep

- Negative self-talk such as "I am sick;" "I am never going to get well;" "my life is ruined"

## 2.  Spirochetes Love Junk Food, Sugar and Processed Foods

Spirochetes love the physiological chaos created by crappy diets of sugar, starches, junk food, artificial sweeteners, salty snacks, high-fat or fried foods, saturated fats (lard, palm oil, beef tallow, butter, palm kernel oil), wheat products, and pastries. These are all meat and potatoes for the spirochetes because they lead to an overloaded liver and inadequate digestion. Illness flourishes on fermented sugars and an acidic environment in the body. Spirochetes will love you and be with you forever if you make them welcome.

## 3.  Spirochetes Play Hide and Seek by Being Labeled As Something Else

If a doctor does not recognize the existence of Lyme disease and treats you for something else, the spirochetes are home free, for nothing is threatening their existence unless by sheer accident. It can be unfortunate or even tragic to be treated for a disease you do not have. For the sake of people who have been to many doctors and gotten all sorts of diagnostic labels, I am including here for reference, some of the labels that Lyme masquerades under. Lyme has been called "the second great imitator" (after syphilis). Unless one suspects Lyme and tests for it, it will probably look like one or more of the following common misdiagnoses (there are too many to list here): Alzheimer's disease; amyotrophic lateral sclerosis (ALS) also known as Lou Gehrig's disease; chronic fatigue immune dysfunction syndrome/chronic fatigue syndrome(CFIDS/CFS); fibromyalgia and Guillain-Barré syndrome; juvenile rheumatoid arthritis; lupus; multiple sclerosis, and syphilis.

Lyme disease can also imitate many psychiatric and neurologic disorders. I agree with Dr. Larry Dossey that these labels constitute voodoo because they lead us to create these very conditions through the power of suggestion. But that is the way the system functions. Someone may tell you that you have attention deficit disorder/attention deficit hyperactivity disorder (ADD/ADHD); anorexia nervosa; dementia; major depression; obsessive-compulsive disorder (OCD); panic attacks; paranoid schizophrenia, or Tourette's syndrome.

### 4. Spirochetes Like to Take Revenge: The Lurking Herx

Spirochetes under attack take their revenge in a "Herxheimer," a temporary worsening of symptoms when you begin a healing program. Sometimes it is hard to distinguish this from the real disease, but it is usually best to continue with clearing toxins until it is over, exercising caution and moderation to keep it from becoming overwhelming or debilitating. Dr. Sarah Myhill lists some of the visible effects of a Herxheimer:[2]

- Strong smelling perspiration or urine

- Metallic taste in the mouth

- Increased thirst

- Nausea
- Headaches
- Feverishness
- Unusual brain sensations
- Dizziness
- Flu-like symptoms
- Cold symptoms such as sneezing, coughing and sore throat
- Fatigue and sleepiness
- Depression, crying, irritability
- Swollen lymph nodes
- Rashes and itching
- Abdominal cramping
- Diarrhea
- Pain in muscles

## What do spirochetes hate?

## Spirochetes (and the biofilms they hide out in) hate everything in this book!

# TWO

# Natural Healing and the Self-Healing Frame of Mind

*But what is quackery?*
*It is commonly an attempt to cure the diseases of a man by addressing his body alone. There is need of a physician who shall minister to both soul and body at once that is, to man.*

Henry David Thoreau

**Attitude:** Self-healing requires a committed mental force to generate momentum and keep it going for however long it takes.

## Rewards of Natural Healing

Many people begin their healing journey with allopathic medicine because they have been taught to do this and also because they are frightened of the changes that are happening in their life. Once the antibiotics stop working it gradually becomes apparent that if you want your life back you have to find other answers.

The wisdom for the path of natural healing comes from the genius for survival within all of us, from trial and error, from knowing what might be too much or too little of something. By keeping things simple, not stressing the brain with complexities and "maybe this, maybe that" worry routines, it is possible to find a protocol that is easy to do for the long haul.

Nietzsche said that we are our own experiments. Natural healing is one of the greatest experiments with ourselves we can do. The rewards are beyond anything we could explain to someone who has not done it. Getting in touch with the ground of one's being is the ultimate prize.

The path to healing body and mind is experimental, experiential, engrossing. The goal is to find a continuum that builds energy and avoids, for the time being, anything that depletes energy. Medical opinions may change from year to year, but the realities of nature remain constant.

# Qualities of the Self-Healer

### 1. Self-Healers Look for Meaning

When Viktor Frankl survived the death camps of World War II he learned that if he took a positive attitude toward unavoidable suffering he could transform it into a triumph, a human achievement. Similarly, if we see in our illness a path to meaning, we can welcome it as a teacher.

### 2. Self-Healing Is an Inward Journey

This journey takes us beyond the narrow limits of medicine, psychology, or theology. Though we may obtain help from others, we are essentially alone with a body and inner being that are crying for us to understand their true reality.

### 3. Self-Healers Eschew Negativity

Self-healers see illness as an initiation into something higher. Illness can teach us to develop higher abilities and skills for dealing with it. Through it we learn to trust our words, thoughts, and deeds as powerful creative forces in our lives. This may be the most important step of all. Hope requires that we give up thoughts of self-hatred or hatred of others. We have to give up the self-punitive attitudes so prevalent in illness. Self-hatred kills.

### 4. Self-Healers Are Proactive and Co-Creative

If we give in to resignation there is little hope for getting well. It sometimes seems as if resignation, rather than disease, is the real adversary. Al Siebert writes that self-healers must find their own strategy for survival. Putting the muscles in motion sends the message to the cells that they are not to resign their life—they still have a will to live. Healing is learning that we can take control of our own life. When there is so much we can do for ourselves, the word is: "save the desperate measures for last!"

### 5. "Please, I'd Rather Do it Myself" or "Me Do it!"

Self-healers make up their own minds. Self-healers determine their own healing path. Self-healers want to discern which voices are authentically true and which are not. We need to have an open mind but also a discerning one. Once the process of self-healing starts, it will unfold according to its own genius: once an intention is known, help seems to come from hidden hands. Blind followers rely on others to know what is best for them. Self-healers are not so quick to follow.

### 6. Engaging in a Self-Healing Routine Is a Worthwhile Thing to Do

Our first duty is to our own body. Sometimes it is only a matter of becoming aware that we are falling into certain patterns, some of which we can easily change. Sometimes we can act "as if," by not letting powerlessness hinder our thinking "fake it 'til you make it." There is nothing more worthwhile than taking back power over our own life.

### 7. Self-Healing Asks for Sacrifice and Awareness

Healing may ask us to make drastic changes in the way we do things. As we grow into this new role, these changes will become the new normal, making many aspects of life more positive. It calls upon us to:

- Venture out of the realm of popular wisdom by feeding mind and soul, as well as body.

- Be patient and persistent for long months or years.

- Make a major, focused commitment to ourselves.

- Know that we do not need to collapse in helplessness—our inner wisdom will tell us what we need to do.

- Be wise enough to know when we are fooling ourselves with false hopes or sabotaging ourselves with false comforts.

- Face possible periods of intense confusion or soul-trying anguish.

- Experience our inner self more deeply, even if it involves facing our worst fears or pains.

- Learn to monitor energy levels, so that we don't crash and have to start all over.

- Give up the desire to return to the old ways that supported us in being sick.

- Put our healing first before anything else.

- Acknowledge and be in touch with the experience of the physical body—we cannot fool ourselves with vague theories or magical thinking.

- Be flexible enough to consider new ideas and be adaptable enough to change if current practices are not working for us.

- Treasure this illness as an opening onto a broader inner life with deeper connection to the great Inner Self.

## Steps to Take

**1. Ask your inner wisdom what you need to make healing happen.**
Make a list and refer to it often. Just thinking about it is a creative act that can bring positive changes.

- What do you lack? What are you crying out for, what nutrients, what mental stimulus, what comfort, what experiences?

- What inner wisdom is seeking expression?

2. **Follow this inner voice and ask it to show you how to:**

- Work with that wise essence within you to find your path.

- Engage with the processes that discourage disease rather than welcome it.

- Use the power of your cosmic mind/being to make unwelcome cells fade away and leave your body.

3. **Write down any suggestions that come to you from your deeper mind or from your dreams.** Try any that seem feasible or attractive to you. Save these images: they may someday point the way for you.

A few simple steps will get you started and keep you on the path:

**A.** **Form the Intention to do whatever it takes to create healing.** This intention comes from inner forces that have become mobilized and focused. Perhaps you are disappointed with answers from conventional sources, perhaps you are tired of suffering, or perhaps you just welcome the challenge.

**B.** **Once you accept that this is an everyday job you will find ways to work these things into a routine.** A different life is not an inferior life. The daily routine becomes less burdensome when you can accept it, do it, and find some satisfaction in the doing.

**C.** **Start anywhere, no matter how simple.** No matter how sick you are, there is always something you can do to start the healing process. Even though you are depleted, can't make it out of the house, can't wash the dishes, can't put sheets on the bed, there is something you can do to start to reverse the energy drain. That might be as insignificant as making a strategic phone call, or buying organic vegetables instead of conventionally-raised vegetables, getting an acupuncture treatment, or making some vegetable juice. The more you build your tower of healing the more psychic energy you will have to apply to the task.

**D. Keep doing it.** Never give up. Don't even question it. Be persistent. Keep doing what you have to, one day at a time, taking little steps if you have to, but taking them—"Little by little, step by step." Always climb back on the upward spiral if through some human weakness you fall off and succumb to a food temptation or a negative thought. Strength will be there. Punishing yourself with recriminations does not help. Your healing will dictate its own pace. Work towards building regular habits of self-healing that are suitable for you.

**E. Go to doctors who believe you can get well.** Al Siebert writes that patients with strong personal power do not respond to placebos or paternalistic doctors. They need to know what is happening and to have a participatory relationship with their doctor. Doctors need to believe everything they tell the patient. Likewise, they need to honor whatever the patient tells them. A doctor should be willing to learn from the patient. A patient who does research into natural healing of his/her own particular illness frequently will have more information than the doctor will, but may want to rely on the doctor for monitoring and support. The rapport between a doctor and patient who are able to learn together contributes enormously to the healing process. Some doctors have such positive energy that just visiting them leaves you with renewed courage and energy. I have found naturopathic doctors to be much more supportive and knowledgeable about Lyme.

**F. Look for Yahoo groups for Lyme disease, chronic fatigue syndrome, and fibromyalgia.** Find people who are doing exactly what you are doing, and who share their stories of success or failure. Do web searches for people who have healed themselves by natural means.

**G. Find someone to cackle with.** This may be one of the most important steps to take. Cackling is a very high and ancient art. It loosens up trapped air bubbles in the system and lifts them into the wide realm of mirth. Cackle is truth in levity: no sacred illusions or artificial modes of thought can coexist with cackle. Join the great sisterhood or brotherhood of truth-cacklers. The antithesis of cackle is to ruminate on your isolation and loneliness.

# THREE

# Build a Strong
# Immune System

**Foundation**: To restore the power that illness has usurped we need to understand basic fundamental processes of the physical body in order to develop a focused and direct biological approach. Any mental-emotional healing benefits from proper function of the physical body.

Ongoing, tightly stressed focus on killing spirochetes with antibiotics is a temporary solution at best because it doesn't make them go away. Dr. Dietrich Klinghardt states that since microbes, given the right circumstances, can change into other microbes, one should give up the idea of combating particular microbes and focus instead on treating the illness as an ecosystem. He suggests that the best approach is to detoxify and learn to live in symbiosis with our microbes. It is pointless to go on, year after year, trying to kill microbes, because these microbes are programmed to survive, no matter what: whether we kill spirochetes with antibiotics or herbs, we will sooner or later have to face the fact that they will return armed to the teeth. Our only option is to simply make them unwelcome in a healthy, restored body.

How do you approach the daunting task of healing yourself of an illness the medical establishment has no answers for? How do you stop making the microbes feel welcome? With dedication, discipline, and determination it is possible to outwit their fierce, but primitive, survival tactics. The personal skills needed for accomplishing this are learnable talents.

# The Th1/Th2 Hypothesis

Immunity is a very complex issue when looked at scientifically. For those of us who are not scientists, it helps to have some idea of what we are working with. The Th1/Th2 hypothesis may or may not be one of the ways immunity works, for "it remains an unproven hypothesis and many of its facets have become untenable."[3] There may be as yet undiscovered inflammatory processes to consider. The current view posits that a healthy immune state would be essentially balanced between "cellular immunity" (Th1) and "humoral immunity"(Th2), although this may be a simplification. For our purposes, it is a good place to start.

Th1 immunity is responsible for reactions to invaders from the environment. Th1 acts primarily against intracellular foreign pathogens such as viruses and bacteria. Th1 pathways offer defense through cytotoxic T lymphocytes, NK cells, macrophages, and monocytes. Th1 immunity depends on normal gut flora for proper functioning. If gut flora is abnormal a decline in Th1 immunity ensues. Lyme would fall primarily in this category, though not totally, since some symptoms arise from the now-malfunctioning body.

Th2 immunity is responsible for issues arising from within the body. Th2 cells are involved in hypersensitivity disorders such as allergies, asthma, eczema, and hay fever, as well as in sclerotic disease and systemic lupus erythematosus. If Th1 immunity fails, Th2 will try to make up for it, but since it is not equipped to do this properly, improperly digested proteins will "leak" into the system, wreaking havoc anywhere they can. When the gut flora is out of balance, the lining of the intestines begins to deteriorate. The results are seen as allergies and food intolerances, headaches, skin conditions, swollen joints, depression, panic attacks or other psychiatric symptoms.

## Nutrients That Modify Th1/ Th2 Response

Melatonin provides a homeostatic link between the brain and the immune system. It has specific high-affinity binding sites on both Th1- and Th2-helper cells. A potent antioxidant, melatonin has been studied as a promising anticancer therapy in combination with low-dose naltrexone (LDN). Melatonin taken at night improves sleep.

Dehydroepiandrosterone (DHEA) is a product of the adrenal glands. DHEA helps the body adapt to stress and may have a function in regulating the immune system. Adaptogen herbs also support the adrenals.

Selenium is an important antioxidant, often lacking in persons with viral, bacterial, and fungal infections. Selenium supplementation enhances Th1 action, improving resistance to invaders from outside.

Zinc deficiency is widespread and results in poor resistance to infections. Zinc is required for the activity of thymulin, a thymic hormone which helps bring T cells to maturity.

Probiotic bacteria such as lactic acid bacteria of the genera *lactobacillus* and *bifidobacterium* can fuel systemic, cell-mediated immunity of the Th1 variety. They improve resistance to cancer and viruses, and may reverse some of the immune deficiencies associated with aging. Probiotics may also help with Th2 conditions such as asthma.

Phytochemicals such as the phytosterols and sterolins are effective for long-term immune benefits. These are found in certain foods (see Chapter 5).

Omega-3 fatty acids, particularly eicosapentaenoic acid (EPA) and docosahexaenoic acid (DHA) from fish oils, have anti-inflammatory properties which protect against heart attack, coronary artery disease, hypertension, kidney nephropathy, inflammatory bowel disease, and inflammatory conditions such as rheumatoid arthritis, multiple sclerosis and type 1 diabetes. They help with morning stiffness, tender joints, and fatigue. Fish oils are effective also for autoimmune conditions.

# Gut and Physiology Syndrome (GAPS)

*And we have made of ourselves living cesspools
and driven doctors to invent names for our diseases.*

Plato

Dr. Majid Ali states that the causes of chronic fatigue, a symptom rather than a disease, are to be found in bowel dysfunction and he states that poor diet and exposure to multiple toxins have left most of us with impaired immunity to all sorts of degenerative conditions. **Since 85% of the immune system resides in the wall of the intestines,** the very foundation of any physical healing program lies in restoring proper gut flora and restoring damaged intestinal walls. Dr. Joseph Mercola adds, "It is becoming increasingly clear that destroying your gut flora with antibiotics and poor diet is a primary factor in rising disease rates. Recent research suggests intestinal inflammation may play a crucial role in the development of certain cancers."[4]

The importance of the gut lining cannot be overstated. Healing it will heal the food intolerances, the headaches, the mental symptoms, and many of the other symptoms of chronic illness. The state of affairs caused by a leaky, overworked, out of balance intestinal system is known as the Gut and Physiology Syndrome (GAPS). GAPS can result in neurological and psychiatric disorders such as depression and obsessive-compulsive disorder, and other problems such as multiple sclerosis, arthritis, asthma, allergies, skin problems, kidney problems, digestive problems, and autoimmune disorders.[5] Without an intact gut lining or proper flora in the intestines, pathogenic forms such as viruses, fungi, worms, and toxins can find their way into the bloodstream and attach to particular proteins, changing them into molecules the immune system cannot recognize.

The molecular similarities between these proteins and the tissues of the central nervous system lead the immune system to attack its own tissues by producing antibodies against them (autoimmune response). An example of this is multiple sclerosis, where the immune system attacks the myelin sheath of the nerves. When the blood brain barrier (BBB) is impaired these undigested particles can make it through to the brain to cause neurological problems and "brain fog." **Until autoimmune diseases are treated as digestive disorders, they will become progressively worse.** It is easy to see that treating Lyme with antibiotics, which can seriously impair the gut lining, is a short-sighted tactic if it leaves one vulnerable to this form of assault.

Other causes of leaky gut are food allergies, overgrowth of candida in the gut, alcohol consumption, infections, parasites, some over-the-counter and prescription drugs, and the proteins (lectins) found in grains and legumes. Candida, for instance, is a major companion of leaky gut. Treating candida involves a front-on dietary change, requiring one to cease eating anything containing sugar or yeast, and to eliminate those foods that cause an autoimmune response or allergic reaction. Once these causes have been removed probiotics, foods high in fiber, fish oil, enzymes, and glutathione will help to heal the gut.

## Sugar is Viagra for Spirochetes, Candida, Cancer, and Viruses

We can deliberately and with great satisfaction frustrate our spirochetes by depriving them of those foods which enliven them. These invaders like everything we can't resist. Our addictions feed them and make them reproduce like crazy. The main offender is sugar, anything made with sugar (such as alcohol), and anything that acts like sugar in the body (aspartame and the like). Since we started eating sugar as babies it is probably more addicting than heroin: it is certainly very difficult to quit.

Most of us have an easily-triggered response to sugar, even if we haven't eaten it for years—sometimes it takes as little as one greasy cookie to start a person back on uncontrolled intake of junk food. Dr. Christine Horner, a breast cancer surgeon says this about sugar:

> To me, sugar has no redeeming value at all, because they found that the more we consume it, the more we're fuelling every single chronic disease . . . In fact, there was a study done about a year ago... and the conclusion was that sugar is a universal mechanism for chronic disease. It kicks up inflammation. It kicks up oxygen free radicals. Those are the two main processes we see that underlie any single chronic disorder, including cancers. It fuels the growth of breast cancers, because glucose is cancer's favorite food. The more you consume, the faster it grows . . . sugar is something that completely knocks out our immune system . . . if you consume a high sugary meal you may knock out your immune system function by as much as 90% for 5 hours afterwards.[6]

When sugar reacts with amino acids a group of compounds called "advanced glycation end products," AGEs are formed. Glycation is a major cause of cell damage leading to illness and faster aging. Therefore it makes sense that restricting AGEs and dietary sugar will prolong life and reduce inflammation and heart disease. Fructose is one of the worst of the sugars, for it promotes growth of fat cells around vital organs, as happens in diabetes and heart disease. High-fructose corn syrup is an ingredient in many processed foods.

# Parasites (The Paparazzi of the Body)

Another reason to avoid sugars and simple carbohydrates is that this is also the diet of choice for parasites. Parasites rob energy from the host. Parasites can be microscopic, like amoeba and giardia, or they can be large like the pinworms, roundworms, tapeworms and flukes found in meat and fish. Since parasites know how to evade detection it is very difficult for T-cells to find them.

The digestive tract is host to about one third of the parasites that live in the body. Others live in the blood, the muscles, the heart, lungs, liver, or brain, where they attach themselves and feed off these organs. We can be unaware of the presence of parasites, since symptoms of infestation often mimic symptoms of other conditions.

Parasites rob us of nutrition and excrete toxic waste products which then circulate in the body. Common symptoms are nausea, diarrhea and abdominal pain, gas and bloating, alternating diarrhea and constipation, bad breath, food allergies, headaches, irritability, fatigue, bowel problems, and stomach ache. Worms can cause weight loss and/or itching around the anus, worms or blood in the stool, or grinding of the teeth at night. The overall effect of parasite infestation is harm to the immune system.

Babesia, a common Lyme co-infection, is a parasite rather than a bacterium, which targets the red blood cells. This malaria-like illness can appear when the immune system is compromised. Ehrlichiosis, another Lyme co-infection, on the other hand, is bacterial: most of its symptoms derive from the immune dysfunction that it causes.

**Note:** If you are dealing with serious gut problems and malabsorption it is best to have some stool testing and other lab work to look for parasites and other invaders. You will probably need to find a good naturopath for this.

## Herbs for Removing Microscopic Parasites

- Black or green walnut hulls
- Olive leaf (oleuropein)
- Pau d'arco bark
- Barberry root
- Shiitake mushroom
- Grapefruit seed extract

## Herbs for Removing Large Parasites

- Wormwood
- Clove bud
- Bitter digestive herbs such as Swedish bitters
- Hulda Clark's parasite removal system: black walnut hull tincture, wormwood capsules, and clove capsules, taken over a couple weeks in graduated amounts. One can buy empty OO capsules and fill them at home with the wormwood and cloves.
- Clarkia tincture

## Fermentation: The Answer to Leaky Gut

In traditional cultures foods were preserved by means of fermentation. This supplied beneficial bacteria for the gut and people stayed healthy. Fermenting provides many more probiotic bacilli than probiotic pills can. Tests have shown that one serving of fermented vegetables could provide the same protection as a whole bottle of high potency probiotics.[7] Recipes for fermented foods are found in Appendix A.

# Food Combining

It is important to eat foods that do not combat each other in the stomach to produce fermentation of undigested food. Some rules of thumb are easy to remember:

- The simplest meal to digest is one in which you eat only one food.

- The fewer foods mixed together the better.

- Oil slows digestion and combines best with fruit and vegetables.

- Since the liver has to process fats, people on a healing program should eliminate all but omega-3 and olive oils (and extra virgin coconut oil if tolerated) and stick to a low-carbohydrate diet.

- Eat all melons alone before eating other foods because they are digested so fast they will ferment when mixed with other foods.

- Honey and molasses eaten with other foods will also cause fermentation and gas.

- It is best to avoid foods that are difficult to digest such as peanuts or dairy products.

## Good Food Combinations

- Protein and leafy greens
- Starch and vegetables
- Oil and leafy greens
- Oil and fruit

## Poor Combinations

- Protein and starch
- Oil and starch
- Fruit and starch

# Glutathione and the Methylation Cycle

**Methylation** is the process by which one molecule, a methyl donor, transfers a methyl group (a carbon atom and 3 hydrogen atoms, or CH3) to another molecule, which then becomes methylated. It is through this process of methylation that the body produces glutathione. Methylation is important because it activates biochemical pathways and reactions which have far-reaching effects:

- It is responsible for production of energy and creatine, carnitine, coenzyme Q10, phosphatidylcholine, and melatonin.

- It is responsible for synthesizing the proteins that make hormones, neurotransmitters, enzymes, and other immune factors. It supplies methyl groups to be attached to DNA molecules. This "reading" of DNA is referred to as "gene expression." If methyl groups are lacking they cannot, for instance, prevent or "silence" the gene overexpression which is characteristic of chronic fatigue syndrome.

- It regulates the sulfur metabolism necessary for detoxification. Sulfur in the diet comes from amino acids such as methionine, cysteine and taurine. People with chronic fatigue often have impaired levels of sulfur metabolites.

- It is involved in the production of myelin and phospholipids in the brain and nervous system.

- It takes part in the metabolism of folic acid.

- It is essential for cell-mediated immune function (T-cells, TH1/TH2 balance, NK cell function) necessary to keep lurking viruses and bacteria from reactivating themselves at will and rampaging through the body. When these cycles are working normally pathogens will be inactive, living "in symbiosis" with the host.

In the diagram below I have taken outlandish liberties with this very complex biochemical reaction. I see this process as an interweaving of parts and processes, metaphorically resembling the Celtic knot, which symbolizes how each is a necessary part of the whole. If one part is missing, the thread unravels. As the normal cycle proceeds, each element of the cycle gives up a methyl group to become the next one in the cycle through the action of enzymes. Activated forms of B12 (methylcobalamin), folate (5-methyl-THF) and B6 (pyridoxyl-5-phosphate) are required for each of these steps. Without a properly functioning methylation cycle this conversion cannot take place.

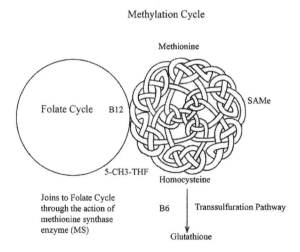

Methylation Cycle

SAMe (s-adenosylmethionine) donates a methyl group to become homocysteine.[8] The methionine synthase enzyme (MS) energizes the activated form of B12 as it combines with folate from the folate cycle to produce methionine. The methylation cycle connects the folate (required for DNA/RNA synthesis) with the glutathione cycle (with its pathway of endogenously produced sulfur required for glutathione synthesis).

Without the action of B-12, folic acid, and methyl donors such as choline or betaine (trimethylglycine), high homocysteine levels can lead to development of a number of serious conditions such as cardiovascular disease, osteoporosis, osteo- and rheumatoid arthritis, multiple sclerosis, Alzheimer's, pregnancy difficulties, renal failure, and type II diabetes. A block in the methylation cycle is also implicated in depression. Improving methylation restores the body's production of serotonin and melatonin, eliminating the need for pharmaceutical drugs for "mental illness."

High homocysteine levels are involved in neurological conditions such as multiple sclerosis. High homocysteine impairs methyl donations for the neurotransmitters necessary for nerve conduction. The transsulfuration pathway provides the sulfur needed for the detox pathways in the liver which bind heavy metals (a factor in both MS and Lyme). The toxicity of the metals interferes with this pathway, stealing the sulfur groups from proteins needed for cell rebuilding and crucial enzyme synthesizing. Heavy metal toxicity thus contributes to neurological damage.

Methyl donors are critical in detoxification. With insufficient methylation the body cannot detoxify sufficiently to protect itself against illnesses such as Lyme and candidiasis. Many foods supply methyl donors.

## Glutathione Deficiency Implicated In Brain Issues

Our defense against invasive illness rests in having a plentiful supply of glutathione in the body. These supplies can be brought down by infections, poor diet, mitochondrial dysfunction, and stress. Lyme disease puts incessant demands on the immune system. Inflammatory and toxic conditions decrease the brain's store of glutathione, manifesting in those strange feelings in the brain, the imbalance, and the dizziness. Lyme toxins can affect and damage brain function or, at the very least, cause distressing cognitive problems (memory, thinking, etc.). Brain inflammation can also result from unrelated causes such as trauma, obesity, exposure to toxic metals and chemicals, and conditions such as diabetes and autoimmune diseases.

Glutathione can keep these brain sensations from happening. It is, therefore, of primary importance to increase glutathione levels and keep the methylation cycle functioning properly.

## Glutathione/Methylation Depletion

Rich van Konynenburg[9] in his study of chronic fatigue syndrome and autism has identified the methylation cycle as a critical element in the immune system.[10] He was able to achieve remarkable results with autistic children after supplementing their diets with methylcobalamin, folinic acid, and trimethylglycine (betaine) in combination with dietary changes and chelation to remove heavy metals. This protocol unblocked the methylation cycle and restored glutathione levels. Without enough glutathione to remove toxins a circular event is created—the supply of B12 is taken over by toxins, leading to further depletion in the glutathione which is attempting to correct this situation. The job of B12 is to form methylcobalamin, one of the two active forms of B12, needed by the enzyme methionine synthase, an essential link in the methylation and folate cycles. Some of the properties of glutathione are:

- It is synthesized by most cells in the body, particularly those in the liver.

- It is the most important antioxidant produced in the body.

- It regulates the important nitric oxide cycle produced by the body from L-arginine, oxygen, and nicotinamide adenine dinucleotide phosphate (NADPH) with the help of nitric oxide synthase (NOS) enzymes. The nitric oxide cycle relaxes the endothelium (inner lining) of the blood vessels and the surrounding smooth muscle, improving blood flow, inhibiting platelet aggregation, and inhibiting the plaque build-up in the endothelium that is responsible for causing atherosclerosis, diabetes, and hypertension.

- It neutralizes heavy metals, carcinogens, and foreign chemicals.

- It is essential for production of lymphocytes, T cells and NK cells, and controls apoptosis or cell death (especially important for cancer cells). Survival rates for wasting, as in AIDS and cancer, are improved by supplementation with glutathione.[11]

- It supports DNA synthesis, repair and enzyme activation.

- It supports the nervous system, the gastrointestinal system and the lungs.

# Restoring the Methylation Cycle

Before beginning any program designed to restore the methylation cycle certain issues must be kept in mind. Dr. Amy Yasko[12] recommends attention to the following:

1. The gastrointestinal system must be able to absorb nutrients from both food and supplements, and be able to remove whatever toxins will be released that way.

2. Over-excitation of the nervous system may make it difficult to tolerate the detoxification process.

3. The person needs to find the appropriate nutritional support

and supplements to rebuild a weakened system and improve overall metabolism.

4. Individual differences need to be understood and addressed, perhaps with supplements.

5. Chronic bacterial infections should be addressed, preferably with natural antimicrobial protocols.

Dr. Sarah Myhill,[13] in her writings on chronic fatigue, suggests the following course of action for restoring the methylation cycle.[14] Please note that this may not be the answer for everyone; some might experience adverse effects.

## For two months take a daily dose of:

Vitamin B12 hydroxycobalamin 5,000 mcg or injections of methylcobalamin 1/2ml or methylcobalamin 1mg sublingually

Folate methyltetrahydrofolate (5MTHF) 800 mg

Pyridoxal 5 phosphate 50 mg twice daily

Glutathione 250 mg daily

Phosphatidyl serine 200 mg once daily

Lecithin (phosphatidyl choline) and phosphatidyl ethanolamine

If you need even more help add:

Tri-methylglycine (also known as betaine, found in beets)

S-adenosyl methionine (SAMe) 400 mg daily

Some people may need to stay on this regimen for quite a long time. It is best to approach this slowly because of possible detoxification symptoms. Once the cycle is working again, it is not so necessary to have the activated B vitamin forms to keep it going—other forms of B12 will do.

Myhill states that eventually this program will lead to:

Improved sleep

Less night-time urination

Return to normal body temperature

Improved blood pressure values

Activation of the immune system against infections

Increased energy without subsequent "crashing"

Elimination of brain fog, with improved cognitive ability and memory

Improvement in hypoglycemia symptoms

Improved tolerance for alcohol

Less pain

Restoration of more normal life, with more calmness

Improved tolerance for heat

Improved tolerance of stress

Shedding of excess weight

## Two Big Herbs for Glutathione Support

Milk-thistle (Silybum marianum)can increase glutathione levels in the liver by up to 35%.

Curcumin (turmeric) also increases tissue glutathione levels.[15]

## Glutathione Precursors or Catalysts

Glutathione does not lend itself to oral administration. In order to produce it in the body and to recycle homocysteine into methionine the body can benefit from supplementation with other key precursors and catalysts such as:

Vitamin B6 in its active form pyridoxal-5-phosphate

Choline and inositol

Dimethylglycine

Melatonin

Magnesium sulfate

Taurine

Minerals molybdenum, magnesium and zinc

Niacinamide

Whey protein isolate[16]

Fish oil

Vitamin D3 or spending time in the sun[17]

Alpha lipoic acid

500 mg. Vitamin C per day raises blood glutathione in healthy adults by up to 50%.[18]

# FOUR

# Good Housekeeping

*And we have made of ourselves living cesspools,*
*and driven doctors to invent names for our diseases.*

Plato

**Reclaim:** restore and revitalize all systems to provide relief from many symptoms, including neurological ones. Improvement can sometimes be rapid and remarkable ("overnight").

## Essential Oils

Essential oils (aromatherapy) are an underground secret for Lyme and many of its symptoms and co-infections. I have found numerous anecdotal reports from individuals who have used various oils to deal directly with their Lyme, in combination with other routines such as a healing diet (no sugar of any kind, or wheat), detoxing routines, and healthier lifestyle.

An essential oil is made by distilling large quantities of a plant to reduce it to its concentrated, powerful essence. These oils are thus much more potent than the simple herbs themselves. Certain oils have long been used against fungi, bacteria, and viruses. These essential oils can damage the cell wall and membrane of these organisms, leading to dissolution of the invading cell and its contents. The advantage of using essential oils in this way is that they are nontoxic, they kill bacteria, they do not lead to resistance as antibiotics do, and they do not leave you with side effects. I have found these oils to have a very energizing effect: they make you feel good!

Lyme has a reputation for being notoriously difficult to treat. One primary factor here is that the bacteria surround themselves with biofilms that enable them to conceal themselves to avoid destruction by antibiotics. In dealing with chronic Lyme, it is the biofilms that really need to be addressed. A study by Nicole Kavanaugh and Katherine Ribbeck analyzed a selection of essential oils for their action against various biofilms. They worked with cassia (*Cinnamomun aromaticum*), clove (*Syzgium aromaticum*), Peru balsam (*Myroxylon balsamum*), red thyme (*Thymus vulgaris*), and tea tree oil (*Melaleuca alternifolia*). Although different types of biofilms reacted to different essential oils, they found that overall the oils were more effective than the antibiotics they compared them to. This led them to conclude that "the species-specific activity of the oils suggests that tailored combinations to target a range of different microbes may be effective against multispecies biofilms."[19] The action of the oils makes it more difficult for the bacteria to hide inside the biofilm and prevents their communication and cooperation with their fellow bacteria.

## Methods of Delivery

1. **Put oils in OO caps for oral consumption**

    A commonly reported method for taking the oils internally is to put them into OO caps with a filler oil such as olive oil. Any oil taken internally needs to be certified as GRAS (generally regarded as safe) by the FDA. Some people create their own mixtures of several oils, sometimes alternating them from day to day. They report taking them up to 4 times or more a day, usually doing this around the clock in the beginning, then tapering off. Capsules are prepared at time of use, for some oils may dissolve the capsules.

    To forestall flare-ups and to combat biofilms the strongest oils to put in a capsule are **oregano** (4 drops), **clove** (3 drops), **thyme** (3 drops). Thyme and clove prevent bacteria from mul-

tiplying. Other oils to try are **cassia** or **cinnamon, melissa, melaleuca, myrrh,** and **eucalyptus blue.**[20]
Oils mixed with carrier oils such as olive may also be dropped under the tongue. Oils may also be added to juice or rice milk instead of being put in capsules.

2. Rectal retention

Though many people report success ingesting the capsules, some say this is not enough. They find rectal retention via suppositories or injection to be the most effective and powerful method of delivery.   Kurt Schnaubelt suggests that the rectal delivery method puts the oils directly into circulation, thus avoiding biotransformation by the liver, allowing them to retain their potency.  He says that when oils are ingested orally they are absorbed into the liver, where they become water-soluble and lose their antibiotic and mucolytic properties.[21]   Any oils used this way should, of course, be pure, organically grown, non-toxic, and non-irritating. Schnaubelt recommends the following oils for general antibiotic use (not specifically for Lyme): mountain savory, *Thymus vulgaris* thymol, and *Oreganum compactum*, 2 or 3 drops per suppository. To make a total of 60 drops per application, add other oils such as *Thymus vulgaris* thuyanol, *Hysop decumbens,* rosemary verbenone, myrtle, or other mild oil. To make the mixture even more powerful, add 1 drop each of cinnamon leaf and cinnamon bark.[22]

For direct injection 30 drops of essential oil mixed with a tablespoon of carrier oil may be injected rectally using a syringe and special applicator tip. Retain this mixture for at least twenty minutes or overnight, if possible. It may take a couple weeks for your body to get used to this procedure. Even if the implant is rejected, you can still benefit from it.

Frankincense, lavender, and lemon oil help clear brain fog and increase energy and immunity.

3. Vaginal retention for candida

Oils will also work for the candida that accompanies chronic Lyme. Common antifungal oils are **melaleuca, blue cypress, lemongrass** (use diluted), **lavender, thyme, mountain savory,** and **melissa.** For vaginal treatment of candida mix up to 30 drops of essential oils with 2 tablespoons of carrier oil and apply to a tampon. Insert and keep it in for up to 8 hours.

4. Topical Application

For neuropathy, oils may be applied to the soles of the feet before bed. Oils applied this way also benefit the entire body. One formula for this is to mix 3 drops each of frankincense, geranium, and lavender. A second formula consists of 3 drops each of geranium, fleabane and cedarwood, along with 2 drops of peppermint. These oils may be applied neat or diluted to the area 3-5 times a day.[23]

## Other Ways To Use Essential Oils

**Massage**: add a few drops of appropriate oils to massage oil.

**Warm compress**: after applying essential oil as desired, cover it with a cloth that has been soaked in hot water and wrung out. To keep the heat in, cover the cloth with a towel or blanket.

**Inhalation**: breathe oils either directly or from a few drops placed in hot water.

**Diffusion into the air**: use a diffuser made for this purpose. Oils such as lavender breathed this way can have a calming effect on emotions.

**Basic safety reminders with essential oils:** Most essential oils may be applied in many ways. Oils that irritate should be diluted with carrier oils such as olive, jojoba, grape seed, or other organic oil. None should be used in the eyes or ears. Oils that need to be diluted are oregano, cinnamon, lemon, orange, clove, eucalyptus, rosemary, peppermint, black pepper, and cassia. If you experience detoxifying reactions, slow your use of the oils either by cutting down on the quantity or adding more carrier oils to them.

# The Liver

Neurons and nerve fibers are vulnerable to toxins caused by infections, trauma, metabolic and degenerative disorders, autoimmune disorders, cancer, and heavy drinking. The Lyme organism itself creates biotoxins that are responsible for neurological problems. Heavy metals such as mercury and lead, man-made environmental chemicals and food additives compound the effects of neurotoxicity. Neurotoxins cause depression, brain fog, memory problems, and insomnia, to mention only a few. Neuropathy (pain, tingling, burning sensation, loss of balance or coordination, and wasting of muscles) is associated with poor digestion and leaky gut.

The liver is a major player in this scenario. A properly functioning liver will improve the methylation cycle and the digestive system. Neurological symptoms may be relieved through care of the liver, attention to the lymph system, and elimination of toxins through the skin with heat therapies.

The liver is located in the upper right portion of the abdomen, just below the rib cage. It receives oxygenated blood from the heart via the hepatic artery, and nutrients from the digestive process via the portal vein. The liver has the task of removing toxic substances from the blood and storing iron, copper, many B-complex vitamins, glycogen, and vitamins A and D. It produces proteins, enzymes, cholesterol, and carbohydrates. The liver becomes overloaded by improperly digested food, drugs, chemotherapy, fats, sugars, preservatives and other foreign chemicals, and by metabolic byproducts of an inefficiently functioning system.

The liver requires a great deal of energy to deal with high toxin loads. A high toxin burden may overload and incapacitate the liver.

This creates a situation similar to a huge traffic jam at rush hour: nothing can go anywhere.

The liver is involved with sugar regulation. Too much sugar affects hormone balance, resulting in poor control over the emotions, anger, low tolerance for frustration, spaciness, mood swings, depression, violent behavior, mental confusion and lack of concentration.

Liver and gall bladder dysfunction show up as fatigue, headaches, insomnia, allergies and food sensitivities, PMS, hypoglycemia, addictions, eating disorders, diabetes, constipation and gas, sclerosis of tissues, frequent night urination, buzzing in the ears, and eye problems such as spots, floaters, dry eyes, and cataracts.

Besides its role in regulation of blood sugar, the liver is also involved in allergies, sleep cycles, mitochondrial function, and thyroid and adrenal hormone cycles.

If the liver is sluggish the entire body will suffer. However, when the liver is working properly almost all the body's processes will be greatly strengthened. Fortunately, the liver responds to self-healing. Once the liver starts to heal, other organs will follow, and the body will slowly begin to return to balance. A properly functioning thyroid depends on a properly functioning liver.

## First Aid for the Liver

**Note:** If there is obstruction of the bile duct, it is desirable to see a doctor before doing any liver therapies.

To start healing the liver, immediately stop intake of the following:

- All alcohol
- Coffee and tobacco
- Too many supplements and over-the-counter drugs
- Meats, fish, and animal fats

- Margarine and processed oils

- Dairy products

- Bread, flour products, cooked grains, and pastries

- Commercial sugar and other sweeteners

- Produce grown with pesticides and herbicides

- Fried foods

- Too much fruit

- Nuts

## Habits That Help the Liver

- Avoid overwork and fatigue.

- Eat in moderation.

- Exercise.

- Practice juice feasting periodically.

- Release anger and worry.

- Avoid emotional stress.

## Herbs to Strengthen the Liver

Turmeric protects and repairs the liver, removing cholesterol by converting it to bile. It is available in capsules or in
bulk in natural food stores and may be placed in "OO" caps
with the "Cap 'M Quik" capsule filler.

Milk thistle (*Silybum marianum*) increases synthesis of glutathione in the liver.

Dandelion is the herb for digestion, liver function, and

treatment of jaundice and is useful for diuresis. It is a tonic, skin cleanser, blood builder, kidney stone dissolver, and mild laxative. The leaves stimulate secretion of stomach juices. The root is a liver tonic and bile releaser, reducing inflammation in the liver and bile duct. It can triple or quadruple the outflow of bile, reducing toxicity in the liver. It has antitumor and cytotoxic properties.

## Other Liver Strengthening Herbs Are:

- •Green leafy vegetables
- •Garlic
- •Aloe vera powder
- •Reishi mushroom (*Ganoderma lucidum*)

## Cholagogue Herbs to Stimulate Production and Flow of Bile:

- Wormwood (*Artemesia absinthium*)
- Oregon grape root
- Artichoke leaf, garden variety
- Barberry root
- Pau d'arco (lapacho or taheebo)
- Yellow dock root
- Bupleurum formula
- Rosemary and sage

## Essential Oils for the Liver

Some essential oils that help in detoxification of the liver are ledum, celery seed, lemon, cardamom, geranium, carrot seed, German chamomile, rosemary and orange. A good blend for the liver is 2 drops German chamomile, 3 drops helichrysum, 10 drops orange, 5 drops rosemary. The gall bladder responds to equal parts Roman chamomile and German chamomile. Oils may also be put in a capsule for ingestion a couple times a day. A few drops of lemon oil taken with water will aid in detoxification processes.

The liver may be soothed by a warm compress placed over it once or twice a day. Mix one part essential oil with four parts carrier oil. Apply 8-10 drops over the liver and cover with a hot, moist hand towel, and then cover that with a dry towel.

## Castor Oil Packs Soothe the Liver

One of the most soothing things for the liver is a castor oil pack. Castor oil packs scare people away because of their gooeyness. However, once you try them for a few days, you may find yourself sleeping better and feeling much lighter in mood. Castor oil contains a unique fatty acid that stimulates the liver, reduces inflammation, and increases lymphatic circulation and NK killer cell production (NK cells deactivate viruses and combat tumors). Packs may also be placed over the thymus gland (which lies under the breastbone) to increase NK cells, and over congested lymph nodes to help move the lymph. These treatments should last for an hour or more, and it is good to do them as often as possible: daily is not too often.

Apply castor oil packs in the evening before bed. Use clean white cotton flannel for the pack (available in fabric shops). Edgar Cayce, the American medical seer, recommended wool flannel, but cotton works just as well. Used cloths may be washed for reuse. If flannel is not available, it is better to use something like a plain paper towel than to skip the application.

1. Place a towel under you to catch any excess oil.

2. Place a heating pad on a flat surface.

3. Turn the heating pad on high.

4. Cover the heating pad with a piece of plastic larger than the flannel. Place a 12" x 12" or smaller piece of flannel on the plastic.

5. Spread evenly about ¼ cup of castor oil in the middle of the flannel—it will spread out as it warms.

6. When everything is warm, pick up the heating pad, the plastic sheet, and oil-soaked flannel. Holding it all together, place it on your abdomen over the liver (or spleen, or thymus).

7. Leave it all on for at least an hour.

8. Do not reuse castor oil.

# Simple Liver (and Lymph) Flushes

Flushing and clearing the liver of stones will improve digestion, allergies, and upper back pain. Most important, it increases energy and wellbeing. I do not favor some of the heroic methods people try for flushing the liver. Gentle liver flushes may be done daily over a short period of time. There is no hurry to get it all done in one fell swoop. For those who wish to do strong liver flushes in a gentler manner, the protocol recommended by Andreas Moritz in *The Liver and Gallbladder Miracle Cleanse* offers possibilities. I also recommend Christopher Hobbs, *Natural Therapy for Your Liver* for suggestions for teas and herbs.

Mark Konlee worked with AIDS patients using a simple, easy, liver and lymph flush. He, reports numerous instances of reversing neuropathy and swollen lymph nodes in as little as fourteen days with his whole lemon drink with olive oil. His reports are based on persons taking this three times a day. He recommends drinking this every morning on an empty stomach for a week. The olive oil will increase production and flow of bile from the liver. The oils from citrus peel are anti-microbial. Lemon juice gets the lymph flowing and reduces swelling of lymph nodes. This drink helps to increase energy and bring new NK and T cells to the lymph nodes from the blood. Whole lemon drink also increases alkalinity as measured in saliva pH.

## Whole Lemon Drink

Start the day with this, and/or have it before meals three times a day.

Mix together in blender:

1/2 of a whole lemon, rind and all

Juice of the other half of the lemon

1 cup of water

1 tablespoon of extra virgin olive oil

2 or more cloves of garlic

Blend for one minute at high speed.

Strain out seeds if you wish.

Konlee found that adding 1 Tbsp. of blackstrap molasses per day also helped to speed up alkalization. He also recommended adding a tablespoon of powdered lecithin for nerve repair.

## Some Natural Ways to Dissolve and Expel Stones

- **Magnesium** supplementation will help clear gallstones, balance excess calcium in the blood and prevent kidney and gall stones. Magnesium makes cholesterol more soluble and easier to remove.

- **Homozon** is a superoxygenated magnesium oxide compound that releases its oxygen through the action of the stomach acids or lemon juice. Besides being an oxygenator, it is a very effective colon-cleansing agent. It can also prevent kidney stones by flushing out excess calcium. Homozon loosens all sorts of toxins and causes frequent eliminations. Although a very effective short-term treatment, it also is difficult to maintain because of the "yuck" factor. Mix a spoonful in water; drink this upon arising. Follow this with lemon juice to dissolve the mineral and release the oxygen. Take Homozon on an empty stomach during the day if you are doing a concentrated cleansing. However, once a day for a week or so will bring about substantial cleansing. Other remedies to consider for stones are:

- **Epsom salts** (magnesium sulfate), taken every morning in small quantities in water, on an empty stomach for a few days

- *Li Dan Pian*, Chinese patent medicine

- Swedish bitters

- Turmeric consumed daily

- Malic acid powder or fresh apple juice with hydrangea and/ or gravel root to soften stones

- Artichoke tincture to dissolve stones

- Lithium carbonate to dissolve uric acids

- Black radish juice every day

- Castor oil taken orally

## Tea for the Liver

**Dr. Randolph Stone's Digestive Tea.** Make this delicious tea in quantity ahead of time to store in the refrigerator for use throughout the day for digestive support.

1 part fenugreek seeds (to reduce intestinal inflammation)

¼ part licorice root (for flavor and spiritual enhancement)

1 part fennel seeds (to reduce gas and cramping)

1 part peppermint leaf (to stimulate digestion, liver, and gallbladder)

Optional: add 1 part of burdock root for increased kidney cleansing or ginger root for improved digestion.

Simmer the first three ingredients for fifteen minutes.

Turn down the heat, add the peppermint, and let it steep for ten minutes.

Other useful teas are nettle, green tea, peppermint (or any other kind of mint), licorice for liver and adrenals, and dandelion root and chicory root as a coffee substitute

## Get the Lymph Moving

Anything that stimulates the lymph will also help digestion and the liver. Anything that helps the liver likewise helps the lymph. The lymph system, which includes the spleen, is responsible for removing and destroying bacterial invaders and transporting digested nutrients from the intestines to the blood stream. It is involved in the formation of NK killer cells to fight invaders. Lymphatic capillaries collect the lymph from all tissues except the central nervous system, and return it to the venous system. Since the lymph does not have a pump like the blood vessels, it relies on the squeezing action of the muscles during physical activity to keep lymph fluid flowing.

Symptoms of swollen or clogged lymph nodes show up in emotional manifestations, "brain fog," insomnia, agitation, obsessiveness, worry, and self-pity. Stagnant lymph is also associated with a number of other symptoms: allergies, many skin conditions, lack of energy and chronic fatigue, parasitic infections, multiple sclerosis, viral and bacterial infections, yeast infections, puffy eyes, cancer , ear and balance problems, arthritis, headaches , formation of cellulite, and excessive sweating.

## Essential Oils for the Lymph

Lemon, frankincense, orange, grapefruit, tangerine, juniper, rosemary, cypress, and myrrh work with the lymph system. Dilute 6-10 drops of one or more of these oils with equal parts of carrier oil and massage this over the lymph glands two or three times a day. A good blend for this is 3 drops of cypress, 1 drop of orange, and 2 drops of grapefruit. Oils may also be applied neat over lymph glands.

Another approach is to diffuse oils into the air for ½ hour every 4-6 hours to stimulate the lymph system.

## Other Topical Applications for Swollen Lymph Glands

- *Phytolacca* (poke root) oil

- Poultice made of mullein leaves steeped for 15 minutes in hot water, drained, and placed on swollen lymph gland

- Castor oil packs or hot packs placed over congested lymph nodes

## Physical Therapies for the Lymph

**Colonics** will facilitate movement of lymph.

**Foot reflexology, hand reflexology, and walking barefoot in wet grass (earthing)** are popular therapies for the lymph. This will stimulate all the acupuncture points in the feet, reflexing to corresponding body parts.

**Exercise** functions like a pump for lymph fluid. **Bouncing on a rebounder** is a very powerful lymph liberator. Thirty minutes a day will keep the lymph moving. Working on the rebounder may also be combined with exercise with oxygen (EWOT), as discussed in Chapter 9.

**Lymphatic massage** will gently move the lymph to the sub-clavian catchment area near the heart for processing. This area must be open before any movement of toxins can happen. The Vodder Manual Lymph Drainage (MLD) method, working with the pulses of the lymph system itself, provides a gentle way to open the lymph flow. The Vodder Method is also one of the most profoundly relaxing massage therapies around.

**Dry skin brushing** of the entire body stimulates all of the acupuncture points and physically pushes the lymph through its channels. This relieves the other organs of elimination such as the kidneys, intestines, lungs, and liver. Brushing minimizes the effects of stress, improves oxygenation of the blood, stimulates brain function and tissue metabolism, and relieves muscular fatigue. The brush should be of a fairly soft natural bristle with a wooden handle so you can reach your back with it. Ten minutes a day is all it takes. Brush towards the heart.

**Ozone saunas, infrared saunas, and other forms of hydrotherapy** directly move the lymph (Chapter 9).

## Primary Herbs for the Lymph and Blood Flow

I have found **Oregon grape root** tincture to be very powerful for lymph cleansing. It is useful for symptom flare-ups. When taking this herb it is necessary to keep the bowel moving in order to eliminate toxins as they are released.

**Venus fly trap** (*Dionaea*) tincture is very active in the lymph. This herb has been shown to reduce the size of lymphoma swellings.

## Other Good Herbs for the Lymph

- Capsicum
- Licorice root
- Ginger root
- Olive leaf
- Red root
- Stillingia root
- Astragalus root
- Mullein leaves
- Bayberry root bark
- Cleavers herb
- Plantain herb
- Echinacea root
- Yarrow flowers
- Garlic bulb
- Xaio Chai Hu Tang
- Hoxsey formula (bloodroot, Oregon grape root, burdock root, red clover, poke root, stillingia, prickly ash bark, buckthorn, *Cascara sagrada*, licorice root)

# Kidney and Bladder

Kidneys are vital in maintaining the life force. They filter out the natural waste products of metabolism and maintain the water balance in the body. Our life processes depend on chemical reactions that create energy. These can occur only in the presence of water. Poorly functioning kidneys can affect the entire balance of the body on a very deep level. Dr. Klinghardt reports that the kidneys and bladder contain the greatest concentration of tissue spirochetes, showing up in symptoms such as cystitis and prostatitis.[24]

Signs of toxicity in the kidneys are difficulties with urination, weak joints, and lower back pain. Signs of poorly functioning kidneys are puffiness under the eyes, weak bones, pain in the knees & lower legs, weak teeth, hair loss or thinning, hormonal changes, reproductive problems, urinary problems such as stones in the bladder, bladder infections, and incontinence.

The adrenal glands are located at the top of each kidney. Kidney disturbances, therefore, can lead to emotional symptoms such as fear, lack of personal power, paranoia, panic attacks, inability to deal with stress, and shaking.

Fighting a disease exhausts the adrenals and can lead to further problems such as elevated cholesterol and triglycerides, skin disorders, carbohydrate cravings, fatigue, and rising homocysteine levels. The methylation cycle becomes unbalanced and levels of the B-vitamins, particularly folic acid and B-12, go down, resulting in depression, joint pain, and gastric reflux. Kidneys need to be functioning to process the added influx of waste material during any cleansing process.

I received the following remarkable comments on my Lyme blog and consider them downright inspiring. Nature does play the major role in our healing if we can work with her on her terms.

## A Communication About Nettles for the Adrenal Glands:

I take stinging nettle capsules every day. I may need to go back to 6 caps/day instead of 3 caps/day, as I seem to need more adrenal support lately. Or I may just get some dried nettle and try some infusions. My brother experienced good relief from joint pain by lightly brushing against fresh nettle leaves 2-3 times a week. This frequency controlled his pain while fresh nettles were available. Anne M., BSN, MSN/IH, RN

Anne M.'s foraging brother John, "forageahead," in lyme-natural-healthcare@yahoogroups.com wrote ( Aug 13, 2010):

> In 2008 I used stinging nettle (*Urtica dioica*) urtication from April to December in about the frequency that bee sting therapy for Lyme disease is recommended. I tried to limit the sting to the itch level. This treatment was not recommended to me by anyone, but from my knowledge of ethnobotany I knew that some tribes used nettle urtication to treat arthritis and rheumatism. My Lyme arthritis was deforming my thumbs, and causing pain in my arms, legs, and back (especially my neck). My ILADS MD said I had fibromyalgia too.
>
> I started out urticating 3 times a week and gradually cut back to 2 or 3 times a month. Then a hard freeze killed all the nettles, that I know of, in the area and I had to stop.

**The results:**

By the end of the first month my fibromyalgia pain had gone way down and my thumbs had lost the deformation and regained full range of motion. During the summer my pain continued to drop (less dramatically than it did the first week). However, my fatigue level did not drop. I lost about 15 pounds without trying (inflammation weight?). The pain has not returned. The pain I am talking about is different from fatigue pain. If I over extend myself I still get a fatigue pain that goes away after adequate rest. This may be 2 to 4 hours of rest or up to 4 days of rest.

I have tried to transplant nettle twice and failed both times. First time the area around my nettle plant pot got sprayed for "weeds". The plant struggled on for 2 months and then died. The 2nd attempt the transplant was not done properly and the roots did not have good soil contact for too long before the defect was corrected. Even then they tried to sprout new shoots that died. Fatigued but not hurting.

Check out John's website: http://www.diningonthewilds.com/dwvfram.htm

## Herbs for Adrenal Stimulation[25]

Licorice root

Stinging nettles

Sarsaparilla root

Seaweeds

Bee pollen

Adaptogens such as:

Rhodiola

Eleuthero (Siberian ginseng)

Astragalus

Ginkgo

Ashwaganda

Schizandra

Licorice

Green tea

Uña de gato

Reishi mushroom extract or capsules

## Essential Oils for the Kidneys

Grapefruit, lemon, geranium. juniper are good oils for the kidneys. A good blend would be 6 drops German chamomile, 6 drops juniper, 2 drops fennel. Put 5 drops of mixture in a capsule and dilute with olive oil. Take a capsule two times a day.

## To Reduce Heavy-Metal Toxicity

- Follow a protocol for restoring glutathione levels and improving the methylation cycle.

- Eat high-quality protein, correct mineral deficiencies, and consume oils such as coconut that protect the nerve sheath.

- Drink lots of water to flush toxins out of the system.

- Decrease the load of heavy metals in the nervous system by eating cilantro as a green vegetable or taking it in a tincture. Note: some people are allergic to cilantro. Eat all the green leafy vegetables you can.

- A very effective derivative of chlorella called NDF or NDF Plus, by Bioray, will cause noticeable herxing from elimination of heavy metals. Though this is fairly expensive, you start with only one drop, and build up to doses of only a few drops, so one bottle should last a while. Follow Dr. Klinghardt's recommendation to follow up with chlorella to make sure the mercury does not just find another place in your body to lodge.

- Increase the levels of oxygen available to neutralize toxins.[26] This can be done through exercise, ozone therapy or other oxygen therapy such as EWOT, exercise with oxygen therapy (see Chapter 9).

# FIVE

# Plant Power

*One-quarter of what you eat keeps you alive.*
*The other three-quarters keep your doctor alive.*

From an ancient Egyptian hieroglyph

**Quality:** Foods that look identical may be vastly different in nutritional properties, depending on how they are raised. Some simple common foods may have powerhouse qualities. This chapter is a brief look "under the hood" of what to look for in foods.

## Sufi Story

Once upon a time a great teacher warned mankind that on a particular date all the water in the world would disappear, to be replaced with new water which would drive people mad. One woman heeded the warning and stored enough water to survive. When the waters dried up she went to her cabin and lived on the water that she had saved. When the new waters appeared below, she found when she went among the people again that they were all thinking and acting in strange ways and had no memory of what happened nor of the warning they had received. When she talked to them she realized that they thought that she herself was mad and they did not understand her. She went back to her cabin. Eventually she became so lonely that she went and drank the new water and became like all the rest. And she forgot about her own water that she had stored, and the townspeople thought that she had miraculously returned to her sanity.

# No More Reckless Eating Habits

The ancient healer Hippocrates said "Let your food be your medicine . . ." Natural healing is based on the principle of "do no harm." This means putting only those things into the body which will promote the functions necessary for living and healing, and refraining from eating anything destructive to the body. A diet that properly sustains us can add enormous energy and impetus to the will to live.

We can take all the herbs in the world or spend the rest of our life on antibiotics, but if we are constantly eating foods that support and maintain our illness, all this will be to no avail. So much can be accomplished through diet that many other (expensive or dangerous) options may not be needed. With any chronic illness, eating needs to become a project, a deliberate choice, rather than the simple satisfaction of hunger in the fastest and easiest or most socially acceptable way. The days of reckless and unconscious eating habits have to come to an end if we want to get well. What we do with food can have a great influence on recovery. Lack of focused attention to diet will most likely result in chronic illness, constant need for doctors, miserable social life, and unpleasant mood states.

## Start with Organic Fruits and Vegetables

Plants need to grow in fertile soil that contains an abundant supply of helpful microbes supplied by decaying organic matter. Soil to which inorganic minerals and synthetic chemicals have been added produces food with far fewer nutrients.

Organically grown foods provide more minerals and trace minerals, phytosterols, phytochemicals, antioxidants and chlorophyll. Organic crops are less contaminated by toxic heavy metals than are conventional crops. The amount of crude protein is lower, but measurement of amino acids, the building blocks of protein, shows the quality of protein to be better. A study by Virginia Worthington shows the astonishing differences in mineral content of organic over conventionally grown food: 500% more iodine; 400% more selenium; 175% more molybdenum; 100% more chromium. Increases in calcium and magnesium are somewhat less dramatic.[27]

# Phytosterols and the Immune System

Sterols are plant oils similar to cholesterol in structure, whose properties are beneficial to the human system. The phytosterols found in most plants are key elements in the prevention and treatment of autoimmune diseases.

- They moderate immune system dysfunction and influence the activity of NK killer cells. Cats with feline leukemia that were given plant sterols were able to maintain their CD4 counts and did not die from their disease. Similar studies showing beneficial effects on the immune system have been made with AIDS patients—sterols and sterolins can dramatically increase the function of T cells.[28]

- Beta-sitosterol, plentiful in the diet of vegetarians, inhibits the growth of colon, breast, and prostate cancer by stopping cell proliferation.

- Sterols can block uptake of cholesterol from the colon, making them useful for regulating cholesterol levels and keeping cholesterol out of the arteries.

- Sterols hinder the inflammatory response and soften the effects of stress. In the treatment of rheumatoid arthritis, phytosterols are anti-inflammatory in the same way that cortisone is, but they do not harm the body.

- They help to regulate sugar levels in diabetes by increasing the levels of circulating insulin.[29]

Plant sterols, called sitosterols, are found most abundantly in cold-pressed plant oils, seeds and nuts. They are present also in all fruits and vegetables, though in smaller amounts. Commercial food oils have most of the phytosterol content removed in order to make the product more appealing to the eye. The phytosterols in cold-pressed olive oil have been shown to reduce cardiovascular disease and some cancers.

One reason to eat plant foods in their natural state is that phytosterols are bound to the fibers of the plant, and vanish with cooking and other food processing. Freezing or boiling vegetables destroys the plant lipids. Sprouting increases phytosterol counts of seeds and nuts, with sprouted sesame seeds and sunflower seeds showing the greatest increases.[30] Since large quantities of phytosterols are required for therapeutic effects, it is a good practice to maximize intake. Rice bran has the highest content of beta sitosterol and beta sitosterolin per cup, followed by sesame seeds and sunflower seeds. Sesame seeds and sunflower seeds may easily be made into delicious milk substitutes (Appendix A). Other sources of phytosterols are buckwheat, almonds and other nuts, corn, peas, barley, fava beans, and olive and flaxseed oil.

# Green Leafy Vegetables Are Super foods

Leafy greens are the number one super food for supporting the methylation cycle and restoring glutathione levels. Leaves are little antennae collecting energy from the sun and converting it through photosynthesis into food energy for animals. Pigments in the leaf absorb various wavelengths of light and store the energy as ATP. When we eat greens and other vegetables raw we take in biophotons, units of light that bring the energy of the sun into our cells. The more biophotons we take in from food, the higher our vibrant energy. Foods highest in nutrition are those that contain the most biophotons.

Different plants absorb different wavelengths of light. The pigment chlorophyll absorbs mainly red, violet, and blue light and reflects green. Other pigments in plants are the carotenoids, flavonoids and quinones, with their various bright colors.

Our very lives depend on the energy we receive when we eat green leaves: dark leafy greens energize on a cellular level and can repair years of poor nutrition. Chlorophyll is "green blood." The similarity to our own blood shows that we are in some miraculous way cousins to the green world. The chlorophyll molecule and the heme (the part of hemoglobin that carries oxygen) of our own blood consist of identical porphyrin rings. The only difference between chlorophyll and hemoglobin is that chlorophyll is built around magnesium rather than iron. The porphyrins in the chlorophyll molecule are necessary for synthesis of the protein portion of the hemoglobin molecule.[31] The "blood" of the green plant stimulates the production of red blood.

## Chlorophyll for Everything [32]

Dr. Norman Shealy considers depression to be the one major illness and that most people die of depression.[33] The other major illness is magnesium deficiency. He considers magnesium deficiency to be at the root of most major diseases, including depression. That magnesium molecule at the center of the chlorophyll molecule could suggest an answer for many of our human ills.

**Chlorophyll plants are cancer fighters.**[34] Chlorophyll and beta carotene in dark green vegetables reduce the possibility of developing various forms of cancer. People who eat more green and yellow vegetables are less likely to die of any kind of cancer.

**Chlorophyll helps regulate digestive problems.** Green vegetables help to heal peptic ulcers and digestive inflammation by regulating the acidity of stomach juices.[35] Chlorophyll alleviates the pain and nausea of ulcers and prevents recurrence of ulcers by checking the digestive action of pepsin.[36] Chlorophyll is a prolific source of digestive enzymes.

**Chlorophyll stimulates tissue repair and inhibits bacteria growth.** Dark green plants have been used throughout history in wound healing and tissue repair. Chlorophyll dries wounds and eliminates odors that may accompany wounds and ulcers. It also speeds healing of burns. Chlorophyll in the diet lessens the possibility of developing skin cancer.

**Chlorophyll is an antipollutant and counters radiation.** The porphyrins in chlorophyll will chelate heavy metals out of the body and help to neutralize toxins and radiation.

**Chlorophyll has a calming effect on the nerves.**

**Chlorophyll neutralizes body odors, including bad breath.**

**Wheatgrass juice** deserves a place of honor among the greens. Wheatgrass is the legacy of Dr. Ann Wigmore, who used it to help people heal from cancer. Since it is better grown, harvested and juiced at home, I will save this for another publication. Wheatgrass may be found in many stores, but usually not in the amounts needed for a determined healing process.

Healing with wheatgrass was first described in the story of Nebuchadnezzar, who suffered a mysterious illness of biblical proportions. I wonder whether he might have been suffering the first known case of Lyme disease. He was forced to get down on his knees and eat grass for seven long years. He was then somehow able to regain his health and his kingdom.

## Spirulina and Chlorella

Brilliant ancient civilizations were built on diets that included daily spirulina. The Mayans built some of the most beautiful temples ever built and developed a calendar more accurate than the one we use today. They plumbed the mysteries of life in their art and architecture. Radar maps of the jungle show that they built a network of narrow waterways for the mass photosynthesis of algae. They used the islands between these narrow, parallel canals for drying the spirulina harvest. The ancient Aztecs, as well, grew spirulina in alkaline lakes and mixed spirulina with the starch of corn as a source of protein.

**Spirulina** is one of the most concentrated foods known. It contains up to 65% protein, three and a half times the protein of beef and eggs (by weight). It contains significant quantities of balanced amino acids, anti-inflammatory and antiproliferative GLA oils, vitamin A, beta carotene and carotenoids, and small quantities of usable B12 cobalamin.

Spirulina is an immune stimulant. It contains a dark blue-green pigment called phycocyanin (1400 mg per 100 g) which imitates the action of the hormone erythropoietin which controls production of red blood cells in the stem cells of the bone marrow. Children whose bone marrow was damaged by radiation at Chernobyl who were given 5 g of spirulina a day were able to recover in six weeks.[37] Spirulina also increases the activity of NK killer cells. [38]

Many people report that spirulina helps to cut down sugar cravings. Just mix a tablespoon in juice or other carrier.

**Chlorella**, another alga, may be as effective in binding bile acids and heavy metals in the intestines as the drug cholestyramine. It also helps increase intracellular reduced glutathione; it repairs nerve damage to some extent; it also contains important nutrients such as B12 and B6; it is good for the immune system and improves bowel flora and alkalinity.

**Use:** add spirulina or chlorella powder to juices and smoothies, sprinkle it on foods, or incorporate it into breads and crackers. You can soon grow accustomed to the unusual flavor. My favorite way of taking spirulina is to add it to raw applesauce.

# Nutritional First Aid Thumbnail Sketch

The right foods can help strengthen normal cells and improve oxygenation of the body. This simplified thumbnail sketch suggests foods to emphasize if you are seeking a higher level of nutrition quickly. These are not the only good foods; this is just a good, very basic place to start.

**Chlorophyll** from green leafy plants, wheatgrass juice, and spirulina

**Beta Carotene** from carrots, baked sweet potatoes, and spirulina

**Anthocyanins** from red and blue fruits such as raspberries and grapes

**Sulfides** from kale and other cruciferous vegetables

**Lycopene** from tomatoes and watermelon

**Phytosterols** from sprouted sesame and sunflower seeds

**EPA oils** from fish for oxygen transport and hindrance of platelet aggregation

**Lignans** from flax seed and burdock root to inhibit absorption of cholesterol

**Limonene** from citrus fruits for immune stimulation and anti-microbial activity

**Turmeric**, anti-inflammatory and liver protective

**Garlic**, potent anti-viral and anti-microbe food

**Green tea** for immune support

**Minerals** from seaweeds (**selenium** is vital)

**Mushrooms** such as reishi and shiitake for immune enhancement

# SIX

# Ground Zero: What Are You Eating These Days?

*If it is made by man, don't eat it.*

Jack LaLanne

*Take care of your body with steadfast fidelity.*
*The soul must see through these eyes alone,*
*and if they are dim, the whole world is clouded.*

Johann Wolfgang von Goethe

**Selection:** It is an encouraging fact that much of the suffering from chronic diseases may be ameliorated by choosing foods that actually heal symptoms and begin to restore the body to a condition of vitality. This starts with the elimination of foods that destroy our natural energy.

A diet designed to restore health would have several goals. Such a diet might:

1. Restore neurological health.

2. Heal a leaky gut, candida, and autoimmune response to stop the body from attacking itself and to improve assimilation of nutrients.

3. Restore the methylation cycle, support the liver, and clear the lymph system.

Some of the most troublesome effects of Lyme are the array of mysterious problems that pop up occasionally. The experience of suddenly feeling bad after eating formerly tolerated foods calls for attention and action: we may have to constantly re-evaluate what we are eating. We need to replace problem foods with others that don't cause problems, and that calls for information. We need to learn to understand the signals our body is giving us. And we need to be strong enough to begin the long and perplexing task of revising our eating preferences.

The information below compares various dietary approaches. One may mix or match or adopt one approach exclusively. The important thing is to do whatever is best for your individual needs. I believe diet is of utmost importance in dealing with chronic illness. I have noticed that when I have been away from home and eating the foods most people eat every day, i.e., cooked, processed foods, the symptoms return.

## What Do You Give Up When You Adopt a Healthy Diet?

Changing to a diet that does not make you sick, provides energy, and helps restore you to a healthy state is a radical change for most people. If you consider in a realistic light how the average diet affects most people, an honest appraisal may lead to some shocking realizations about how it has kept us enslaved and controlled. A change to a better diet would call for some sacrifices. This is what you would have to give up:

1. Cravings: no more trips in the middle of the night to find a Twinkie to comfort you until morning

2. Stumbling over your own feet, reeling around like you are drunk and dizzy from the excitotoxins in processed foods

3. Disgusting antacids, heartburn, or acid reflux "disease" from acid-forming foods and a damaged gut lining

4. Side effects from addictions, post-sugar lunacy, mood swings, depression, and chronic anxiety

5. That hollow, dreadful suspicion that you don't really know exactly what you are eating or what is in it, that secret, unacknowledged fear that something you eat will one day give you cancer or force you to go on kidney dialysis or worse

6. Surly disposition, "choleric" temperament, or uncontrollable rages caused by a plugged up liver

7. Fast food hell and the burden of indigestible food weighing heavily in your stomach

8. Halitosis from putrid matter in the intestines

9. Constipation and laxatives and cathartics

10. Excess weight, premature aging, and facial wrinkles

# Reversing Neuropathy: Where Is Betty Crocker When You Need Her?

Many Lyme people experience symptoms suggestive of multiple sclerosis. Is this a case of "a rose by any other name?" Who knows for sure? There is no single test that will specifically diagnose multiple sclerosis. It would seem to make sense that similar physiological processes may be happening and it would not hurt to look into how MS people deal with their symptoms.[39] When I was experiencing some of these symptoms, I investigated the MS and the Paleolithic diets and made some fortunate changes: I eliminated foods forbidden in either of these diets, and started giving myself B12 shots every day. I believe the **main culprit in my tremors was soy,** a legume. I was eating tofu instead of meat and drinking soy milk like there was no tomorrow. When I eliminated all soy products the tremors improved overnight. The B12 shots restored some of my lost mental function. When I started using extra-virgin coconut oil every day, nerve symptoms got even better.

Just for reference, here are some of the symptoms associated with multiple sclerosis:

Tremors of hands, arms, and legs

Paresthesias (pins and needles) and tingling of hands, feet, and face

Clumsiness, poor coordination, problems with balance

Unsteady gait

Flashing lights, eye events and problems

Blurred vision, double vision

Red-green color distortion

Eye pain, blindness in one eye

Rapid involuntary eye movement

Partial vision loss

Muscle weakness or stiffness

Pain

Loss of feeling

Numbness

Mental problems with cognition, concentration, attention, memory and judgment

Speech disorders, slurred speech

Bladder problems such as incontinence

Emotional changes

Paralysis

Impotence

**The MS diet** prescribed by many doctors is very similar to the Paleolithic diet. The basic difference between the two diets is that the MS diet forbids eggs. People with MS use essential fatty acids (EFAs) to arrest or slow the deterioration of nerve fibers. They also avoid the harmful fats[40] found in margarine (unless non-hydroge-nated), partially hydrogenated oils, shortening, deep fried foods, commercially refined oils (all, including "extra virgin" unless ex-plicitly stated to be unrefined), and mayonnaise.

# Healthy Fats and Magnesium for Nerve Health

To control troubling neurological symptoms, avoid all but

- Monounsaturated oils (extra virgin olive oil)

- Polyunsaturated oils (unrefined sunflower and safflower oil)

- Omega-3 essential fatty acids from fish and flax oil

The all-important **omega-3 fatty acids** must be obtained through the diet because they cannot be made by the human body. Omega-3 fatty acids have a role in preventing heart disease, rheu-matoid arthritis, and cancer. They also help to improve mood and memory. Fresh, oily, cold-water fish is the richest source of ome-ga-3, particularly EPA (eicosapentaenoic acid) and DHA (docosa-hexaenoic acid). Those from plant sources are in the form of ALA (alpha linolenic acid). Seeds are one of the best sources of omega-3 from plants. Seeds are about 1/3 fat, most of which is unsaturated fat. Some research indicates, however, that ratios of excessive lev-els of omega-6 found with omega-3 in flax seeds may increase the possibility of contracting a number of other diseases.

During periods of cleansing, omega-3 fish oils may be taken up to four times a day. A regular daily dose is twice a day. Of fish foods, mackerel, salmon, and sardines are highest in omega-3. Of plant foods walnuts and flax seeds are as high as or higher than the fish sources.

**Organic "Extra Virgin Coconut Oil"** appears to be a miracle food for many neurological problems. Coconuts are nature's most abundant source of medium chain fatty acids and are the source for lauric acid, caprylic acid, and other antimicrobials. Most com-mercial vegetable oils are long chain fatty acids, which are much more difficult to digest. Some of the medium chain triglycerides in coconut oil are used in the liver to produce energy, while others are converted into ketones. Ketones are a powerful form of energy needed particularly by the brain, the heart, and other tissues. They activate certain proteins used in brain cell preservation, restoration, and growth.

Coconut oil supports the immune system.[41] It improves the absorption of B vitamins, vitamins A, D, E, K, beta-carotene, CoQ10 and other fat soluble nutrients, the minerals calcium and magnesium, and some amino acids.[42] Coconut balances blood sugar levels, thus reversing the underlying cause of diabetes.[43] Coconut oil can prevent and even reverse liver disease caused by various toxic agents such as alcohol, bacteria, drugs, and chemicals.[44] It protects other organs in the same way as well.

**Magnesium** is a critical nutrient for neurological issues. Deficiencies in magnesium are a factor in constipation, muscle cramps, chronic fatigue, heart attacks, asthma, kidney stones, PMS, cravings for sugar and chocolate, intestinal cramps, and restless leg syndrome. Magnesium is involved in over 300 enzyme actions and is necessary for production of energy. It relaxes muscles and is involved in the production of serotonin. Again, the best consistent source of magnesium is green plants and green juice. Other foods high in magnesium are cocoa beans, seeds, nuts and whole grains.

## Good Food Sources of Magnesium

|  | Mg/100 gm |
| --- | --- |
| Pumpkin and squash seeds | 534 |
| Brazil nuts | 376 |
| Sesame seeds | 356 |
| Sunflower seeds | 325 |
| Almonds | 286 |

# Garden of Eden: No Pizza Parlors or Donut Shops

The Paleolithic diet reconstructs the diet of our early ancestors, and is based on the premise that we are not much different physiologically from our forebears, for it takes many thousands of years to adapt to cultural dietary changes. Our species has not had time to develop the enzymes necessary to digest many of the unnatural foods and chemicals we eat these days. These relatively recently introduced foods appear to be making us sick. Any food adopted after the cultivation of grain began 10,000 years ago is most probably very difficult to digest and assimilate.

The early diet consisted of foods eaten just as they came from nature, foods that could be easily plucked from bushes or trees or dug from the ground. This was supplemented with the occasional lean wild game. Early humans did not eat the grains and other foods which now contribute to food sensitivities and autoimmune responses.

The introduction of grains, beans and potatoes in agriculture were game changers in the human diet, for they changed the way we live on the earth. They are too toxic to be eaten raw, for they contain enzyme blockers. They must be cooked (or sprouted, in the case of grains and beans) completely to eliminate the toxins and become digestible. They are a source of rapidly available, high glycemic carbohydrate and are poor sources of vitamins, minerals, antioxidants and phytosterols.

Our present diet consists of high protein, high fat and high-carbohydrate over-nutrition. Can we live with a diet like this and hope to cope with the dizziness and cognitive problems caused by a blood-brain barrier that is so damaged that it reacts to everything we eat?

Study of the Paleolithic diet is valuable, if only because it spells out what we should not eat. These guidelines are very similar to those of the multiple sclerosis diet. Avoidance of problem foods has led to many reports of autoimmune diseases being improved or healed altogether. The elements of the Paleolithic diet may seem

restrictive and unfamiliar, but strict interpretation does not always allow for individual differences. Pay particular attention to
soy, which Charlotte Gerson says is poison, and to sugar, which
others have suggested will be the downfall of western civilization.
Reverting to the simplicity of the Paleolithic diet or the MS diet has
some very beneficial effects:

Neurological problems improve.

Blood sugar stabilizes.

Stored fat is burned up.

Allergies become less evident.

Energy remains constant throughout the day.

Inflammation is reduced.

Sleep improves.

Skin becomes clearer.

## Foods to Avoid Altogether

On the Paleolithic diet, and likewise on the MS diet, the foods to
avoid would be:

- Cereal grains and gluten, including  barley, corn (including
  corn syrup), millet, oats, rice, rye, sorghum, wheat, and wild
  rice

- Legumes, including all beans and peas, snow peas, black-
  eyed peas, soybeans and all soybean products, chickpeas and
  lentils, peanuts and peanut butter

- Starchy tubers such as potatoes and tapioca

- Dairy foods, including milk, butter, and processed dairy
  foods (however, whey protein and cultured milk products
  produced through natural fermentation, along with colos-
  trum and transfer factors from milk are good for therapeutic
  use)

- Addictive high-stimulus, manufactured foods containing sugar, white flour products and solid fats

- Food additives or excitotoxins (their name says it all) such as aspartame and chemicals added to fast foods to make them addictive

- Salty foods such as chips and other commercial salty snacks, smoked, dried, and salted fish and meat, most salted canned meats and fish (although you can soak them to remove the salt)

- Fatty red meats from commercially raised beef, and dark poultry meat

- Sugar, including "evaporated cane juice," agave, honey, molasses, maple syrup, high fructose corn syrup, all candy, soft drinks, milk sugar

- Alcoholic beverages

- Dried fruits

- Anything that acts like sugar in your body such as manufactured sugar substitutes

- Canned, bottled, and freshly squeezed fruit drinks (which have a much higher glycemic index than the fruit alone)

- Diet sodas

- Aspartame (a heavy-duty nerve toxin)

## Other items to consider eliminating are:

- Coffee and tobacco

- Too many supplements and over-the-counter drugs

- Produce that has been grown with pesticides and herbicides

- Fried foods

# Healing Leaky Gut with Food

### Strengthen the Blood Brain Barrier (BBB) with Bioflavonoids

Leaky gut permits improperly digested food to invade a damaged blood brain barrier. Maintaining the blood-brain barrier is essential for minimizing some of the troubling brain manifestations of Lyme. Bioflavonoids are anti-inflammatories that help protect the blood brain barrier. Good sources of bioflavonoids are:

- Fruits and fruit rinds, especially citrus fruits

- Ginkgo biloba

- Red onions

- Parsley

- White and green tea

- Red wine

- Blueberries, cherries, blackberries, purple grape skins and seeds, mulberries, cranberries, and clingstone peaches

- Dark chocolate (with a cocoa content of seventy percent or greater)

- Whole lemon drink taken every day

- Supplements derived from the bark and needles of pine trees

Avoid fats such as oleic acid (rendered tallow), trans-fatty acids (man-made fats) and saturated (hard) fats. The most damaging fats for the brain are the hard fats found in fatty beef, gravy, cheese, and many commercial baked goods.

## Foods Beneficial For Leaky Gut

Fiber is number one in healing the gut. Chia seeds are a good source of fiber and may be eaten by themselves or added as is to other foods. Pumpkin and sunflower seeds are a good non-sugar snack.

Their high levels of omega-3 fatty acids combat inflammation and support the thyroid. Pumpkin seeds may be added to smoothies and salads.

Fermented foods and probiotics are crucial in restoring and maintaining healthy intestinal flora. Particularly valuable are *Lactobacillus, Bifidus,* and *Saccharomyces boulardi.* If you buy fermented milk products such as yogurt, avoid those that contain added sugar. The probiotics in fermented foods are many times more powerful than store-bought capsules. Fermented foods are easy to make and easy to eat. Try fermented beet juice, raw sauerkraut or fermented cabbage juice (Appendix B).

**Cabbage** in the form of coleslaw, raw sauerkraut or cabbage juice helps heal leaky gut.

**Raw applesauce** makes a good breakfast every morning if you can tolerate the sugar in apples. Raw applesauce will eventually normalize bowel movements that have been disrupted or destroyed by antibiotics.

**Aloe vera powder**, taken throughout the day, will flush and soothe the intestines while cleansing the lymph system. Aloe powder is a better choice than aloe juice, since the juice may contain preservatives.

**Extra virgin coconut oil** is a medium chain fatty acid rather than a monounsaturated fatty acid like olive oil. Many people are consuming coconut oil every day and reporting improvement in many symptoms, particularly neurological ones. The usual recommended dose is two or three tablespoons per day. It is easily incorporated into other foods. Since it does not break down with heat, it can be used in cooking and in sauces over steamed vegetables.

**Raw garlic**, up to 16 fresh cloves a day,[46] is a great detoxifier and anti-bacterial. It helps restore the good bacteria in the digestive tract and drives parasites away. Garlic cloves may be added to fresh juices or crushed and added to smoothies or water. Garlic should not be taken on an empty stomach.

**Onions** have similar benefits as garlic.

**Flaxseed, bentonite clay from a nontoxic source, slippery elm inner bark, fennel seed, and activated charcoal** are soothing to the intestines.

**Fructooligosaccharides** promote the growth of good intestinal flora. These are found in bananas, Jerusalem artichokes, onions, asparagus, and garlic.

**Ginger** may be used liberally to quickly aid digestion and relieve bloating. Grated fresh ginger root with lemon makes a pleasant tea.

**Seaweed** is a primary food for the thyroid gland because of its iodine content. The minerals in seaweed help to neutralize and remove toxins and heavy metals from the body. Sprinkle kelp powder on food instead of iodized salt. Oriental food stores carry a variety of seaweeds for cooking.

**Olive oil and olive leaf extract** contain oleuropein, a potent anti-fungal. It also helps to keep blood sugar levels down.

**Lime and lemon juices** are good digestive aids. Whole lemon drink will revitalize the liver and immune system.

# Forbidden Foods for Candida

Candida feeds on sugars and yeast. Therefore, the list of specific foods forbidden while treating candida reads like a list of our most addictive foods. I include it again for emphasis:

> **Sugar**, all forms
>
> **Corn**, closely related to sugar and an inflammatory food in itself
>
> **Refined carbohydrates** such as bread, pasta, cereals and other flour concoctions (wheat is associated with arthritis and bloating)
>
> **Commercial dairy products** because of lactose (sugar) content and allergenic potential. Commercial milk may also contain residual antibiotics which can feed the intestinal

flora that promote growth of candida.

**Alcoholic beverages**

**Peanuts** because of possible high yeast or mold content

**Caffeine** because of its effects on heart, nervous system, and joints

# Eat to Restore the Methylation Cycle

The proper foods can supply glutathione and strengthen the immune system. Restoring glutathione with food is a long-term project.

## Methyl Donors and Glutathione in Foods

Methyl donors are found in foods such as **beets, blackstrap molasses, and wheat germ.** Beets are a primary source of betaine, a crucial link in the methylation cycle. Other foods containing betaine are **capsicum, cranberry, red onion skins and red bell peppers**. Of these, beets would seem to be the easiest to consume in quantity.

**Chlorophyll-rich foods** raise glutathione levels. All green plants provide chlorophyll.

**Cruciferous vegetables** supply the sulfide important for the methylation cycle. Choose **broccoli, Brussels sprouts, cabbage, cauliflower, collards, kale, kohlrabi, mustard greens, radish, rutabaga, turnip, or watercress.** Three-day-old broccoli and cauliflower sprouts contain 10-100 times more anticarcinogenic and antimutagenic compounds than the mature plants.[47]

Per serving, **asparagus** contains more glutathione than all other fruits and vegetables analyzed to date.[48] The following have the highest glutathione content compared to other vegetables. It should be noted that these foods can lose substantial amounts of their glutathione when they are cooked, but not when eaten raw:

Asparagus

Avocadoes

Squash

Okra

Cauliflower

Broccoli

Potatoes

Spinach

Walnuts

Garlic

Beets

Pine nuts

Collard greens

Raw tomatoes

# Love Your Liver with Food

A properly functioning liver plays an important role in maintaining the methylation cycle. Since the liver has to process fats, anyone on a healing program should temporarily eliminate all but **olive oil and omega-3 oils** in order not to stress the liver.

Eat a **low carbohydrate diet** until the liver improves. Carbohydrates (grains and sugars) are hard on the liver. Low-carbohydrate vegetables have the least impact on the liver. If you are really in trouble, start with the vegetables which are lowest in carbohydrates, then gradually expand to include the other vegetables. Carbohydrates are lowest in (alphabetical order):

Asparagus

Green leafy vegetables: chard, wild greens, romaine, collards, kale, spinach, parsley

Bean sprouts

Cabbage family: broccoli, cabbage, cauliflower

Celery

Cucumber

Garlic

Mushrooms

Radish

Raw corn

Summer squash and zucchini

Neurotoxins respond quickly to foods that can clear the liver. Special foods for the liver:

**Fresh burdock root and juice** offer a quick, effective, and gentle way to relieve and soothe the liver, cleansing kidney and liver simultaneously. It is easy to juice the fresh root with other vegetable juices on a daily basis.

**Beets and beet greens, raw borscht, and red chard** are medicine for the liver. Beets help reduce fat in the liver and protect it against damage from chemicals and alcohol. The red coloring agent, betaine, brings this about, making beets a primary treatment for liver ailments. The "beet cure," eating beets, cooked or raw and drinking beet juice, is a very effective support for many diseases. Mark Konlee reports 90-100% declines in viral load in two persons with hepatitis C who ate 1 pound of beets a day (raw, cooked, or juiced) along with their other routines. Beets help to form red blood cells. Greek mythology tells us that the goddess Aphrodite maintained her beauty by eating beets.

**Black radish** is considered to be as potent as beets for treatment of the liver. Begin with small quantities.

The liver loves **green leafy plants** such as spinach, kale, romaine, and collards, as well as juice from dandelion, chickweed and other wild herbs. Freshly juiced kale, collards, or other strong greens, watered down with other juices such as cucumber and carrot, will stimulate flow of bile. One of the best wild greens for the liver is nettles, steamed as a vegetable in the spring.

**Carrot juice** is a tonic for the liver.

The liver loves **lemon, garlic, and Jerusalem artichoke juice. Whole lemon drink**, taken on empty stomach before meals is a good tonic for the liver and the immune system. It may stop liver pain, reduce dizziness and brain fog, decrease depression, and shrink swollen lymph nodes.

## Food for the Lymph System

Almost any foods that are good for the liver will also keep the lymph system moving. Particularly beneficial are the **whole lemon drink, burdock root, black radish or beet juice, beets and beet greens**, and **aloe vera powder**. Additional help for the lymph comes from:

**Drinking plenty of filtered water**, especially ozonated water, up to 8 glasses a day

**Raw fruits, especially lemons**
Some fruits such as apples and grapes, sweet citrus fruits, and watermelon, help the lymph, but the sugar in them may make them counter-productive for people who need to reduce sugar intake. Eat low-sugar fruits such as berries.

## Food for the Kidneys

While all the above foods are good for the kidneys, some foods are particularly beneficial for the kidneys:

Burdock and burdock juice or tea, sipped during the day

Black cherries and black cherry concentrate

Asparagus

Fresh parsley juice

Ginger

Nettles and other wild greens

Cranberries and cranberry juice

Citrus, especially lemons

Watermelon (if you can tolerate the sugar content)

Cucumber

## Summary: Basic Food Changes to Start With

Highly processed foods are taken for granted by most people these days. Those who feel it is better to eat higher energy foods generally eliminate these chemically modified foods and cut way down on high carbohydrate foods. Foods to eliminate and replace are:

- **High-fat animal products from commercially raised animals**: meat from grain-fed animals contains more fats of the wrong kind. Grains fed to humans also produce similar "marbling" effects in body fats.
- **Grains and sugars**: they tend to cause allergies in sensitive individuals. Try stevia, an herb which, with a little imagination, can substitute for sugar. It contains good phytonutrients and trace minerals. It does not have the side effects of sugar and it has no calories. Xylitol and other sugar alcohols do not act like sugar in the body but taste like sugar. They do seem to cause diarrhea, though.
- **All manufactured fake sugars** such as aspartame (Nutra-Sweet and Equal), sucralose (Splenda), and saccharin (Sweet'N Low).
- Replace **soft drinks, fruit juices and pasteurized milk** with pure, clean water or almond, coconut, or seed milks.
- **Nearly all processed fats**, especially the trans fats, as they disrupt communication between nerve cells.
- **All junk food, all processed foods, artificial colors, flavors and preservatives.**
- **Beans, particularly soy products**

# SEVEN

# Living High with Food

*The doctor of today does not become the dietician of tomorrow;
the dietician of today will become the doctor of tomorrow.*

Dr. Alexis Carrel

No amount of surgery, pills, therapy, or money can keep
us well. Only a desire and willingness to learn more
about nature, and to embrace her laws, can do so. This
means that we must eat foods such as sprouts, greens,
wheatgrass, fruits and vegetables, with all their vital
nutrients intact—in their natural, living state.

Ann Wigmore [49]

**Energize.** Life force increases with every positive thing we do.
Eating a high-energy natural diet stirs the creative intelligence of
healing.

## Apologia

My intention in this section is not to try to tell people what to eat.
I know that changes usually come slowly and that most individuals
have personal preferences that need to be accommodated. It is not
hard to notice that each new year brings with it new dietary theories, so it can get very confusing. I would simply encourage people

who are trying to get well to find the best, most healing diet to keep cravings in check, and to avoid mass-produced denatured foods.

# Energy

Recovery of wellbeing requires an ongoing and cumulative wave of energy. To surf this wave we need to learn what gives momentum and what deflates our being. A constant flow of energy becomes the wind that keeps us on course. When we have insufficient energy we go nowhere.

A circular relationship exists between illness and energy. Lack of vitality contributes to development of illness and illness leads to further depletion of vital energy. This ultimately results in dissociation of body and soul, and alienation from life. Depressed and bored, we don't know who we are or how we function in the world. It is almost as if we have given away the best and most exciting part of ourselves to an unknown dictator-in-chief to squander as he pleases. We lose our personal power, the very foundation of the will to survive.

Illness cannot coexist with high energy in the body. Physical healing requires repair of everything about our body, all organ systems, all digestive processes, and all mental imbalances. This will create the physical and personal energy to throw off illness. More energy is available to us than most humans can tolerate. There is enough to heal all of us.

Any increase in energy will benefit the spirit: likewise, cultivating the spirit will produce energy. Increased energy improves the function of the physical organs. Where sufficient energy exists, the spirit remains in charge and a state of balance is possible. According to Chinese medicine, energy rises as consciousness rises. According to yogic thought, energy is consciousness. Energy is necessary for the blood to move. Vitality is the very foundation of the immune system. Where the energy goes, the blood flows.

# Acid-Alkaline Balance

A healing diet would increase the alkalinity of the body. Acid conditions underlie many health problems. Acids are compounds that release hydrogen into a solution, whereas alkalis are compounds that remove hydrogen from a solution. Overly acid conditions in the body can lead to muscle contractibility impairment, retention of extra sodium, drowsiness, and other unwelcome changes. **Acidity is accompanied by a deficiency of oxygen in the blood, leading to a situation of chronic fatigue.** Acidity is often the cause of the **muscle cramps** experienced by many Lyme people. Acidification of the blood is a major contributor to conditions such as osteoporosis, nervous disorders, kidney stones, chronic fatigue, gout, arthritis, and dental decay.

Excess acidity causes mucus formation in the body which puts out a welcome mat for pathogens, inviting disease. Dr. John Christopher, the noted herbalist, was a proponent of a high-energy mucusless diet of mostly raw foods. He said if you planted some raw rice and some cooked rice side by side, only the raw rice would have enough vitality to sprout and grow, whereas the cooked rice would rot.

## Acidity can be caused by:

Poor elimination of toxins from the body

An acidifying diet

Stress, anxiety, fear, and other emotional distress

Poor digestion

Metabolic factors

Improperly functioning kidneys and lungs

Heavy metal poisoning

Infections and toxicity from diseases

Prescription or recreational drugs and some supplements

High fat diet

Smoking and alcohol

Poor assimilation of vital nutrients from food

A proper balance between acid and alkaline is necessary because many functions depend upon a particular pH existing in a particular part of the body. Ninety per cent of the calories of the standard American diet come from acidifying foods. Hunter-gatherers, on the other hand, had a high potassium balance from eating a largely plant-based diet. The Gerson diet of raw juices emphasizes potassium to counterbalance the excess of salt in the modern diet. Restoring the normal pH often leads to dramatic improvements in symptoms.

Foods that produce an alkaline ash (are alkaline forming) in the body contain the minerals that form alkaline compounds: calcium, magnesium, and potassium. These minerals neutralize acid forming foods. Higher intake of potassium helps cells release toxins for removal by kidneys and lungs.

## The best alkalizing foods are:

- Most fruits and vegetables, except for legumes
- Raw goat milk
- Goat whey
- Quinoa
- Millet
- Dried dates
- Dried figs
- Dulse seaweed

Acid ash (acid forming) foods contain minerals that produce

acid compounds: chlorine, phosphorus and sulfur. These remain in the body as sulfuric and phosphoric acids.

## High phosphorus, acid ash foods are:

- Meats, bacon and sausage, seafood

- Grains, except for millet

- Pasteurized dairy products

- Cage-raised commercial eggs

- Fried foods

- Legumes

- Fruits that contain either oxalic or benzoic acid such as plums, cranberries, rhubarb and sour cherries

- Most fats

- Chocolate, carob, mustard, coffee, tea, soft drinks, unbuffered vitamin C

- Sugar, nuts, corn oil and corn syrup

- Acid fruits such as tomatoes or citrus fruits, which normally are alkaline-forming, may be acid forming for persons with low stomach acid or low thyroid activity.

## Restore Proper Alkalinity.

Raw foods, being more alkaline, improve the body's acid/alkaline balance. Fresh live fruit and vegetables and their juices, especially lemon juice and foods such as avocados and raw sauerkraut contribute to alkalinity. Pectin from foods such as citrus rinds and apple sauce will assist in assimilation of the fatty acids responsible for acidity. Lemons are popularly assumed to be acidic because of their tartness, but in reality, their high potassium content makes them one of the best alkalizers. These foods also ensure adequate intake of minerals, especially magnesium, potassium and zinc. Greens are the highest food sources of potassium. The following table lists alkalizing greens highest in potassium.[50] Alkalizing greens have a high potassium, low phosphorus ratio.

| Per 100 g | Potassium mg | Calcium mg | Phosphorus mg |
|---|---|---|---|
| Dulse (seaweed) | 8,100 | 567 | 270 |
| Kelp (seaweed) | 5,273 | 800 | 240 |
| Nettle, dried | 3,450 | 2970 | 680 |
| Irish Moss (seaweed) | 2,844 | 885 | 157 |
| Lambs Quarter | 684 | 309 | 72 |
| Amaranth | 617 | 448 | 67 |
| Beet greens | 570 | 119 | 40 |
| Chard | 550 | 88 | 39 |
| Nori (seaweed) | 510 | 260 | |
| Spinach | 470 | 93 | 51 |
| Mallow | 410 | 249 | 69 |
| Dandelion | 397 | 187 | 66 |

| | | | |
|---|---|---|---|
| Kale | 378 | 179 | 73 |
| Dock | 338 | 66 | 41 |
| Watercress | 282 | 151 | 54 |
| Chickweed | 243 | 160 | 49 |
| Cabbage | 233 | 49 | 29 |
| Plantain | 227 | 184 | 52 |
| Burdock root | 180 | 50 | 58 |
| Purslane | | 103 | 39 |
| Alaria (seaweed) | | 1300 | 260 |

## Some Other Foods with High Potassium Content (shown in mg) [51]

| | | |
|---|---|---|
| Avocado | 1 medium | 1360 |
| Tomato sauce | 1 cup | 909 |
| Dried apricots | ½ cup | 898 |
| Potatoes | 1 medium | 782 |
| Cantaloupe | ½ medium | 782 |
| Papaya | 1 medium | 781 |
| Prune juice | 1 cup | 707 |
| Figs, dried | 5 medium | 666 |

| Lima beans | ½ cup | 582 |
| Parsnips | 1 cup | 573 |
| Pumpkin cooked | 1 cup | 564 |
| Watermelon | 10" slice | 559 |
| Raisins | ½ cup | 545 |
| Kiwi fruit | 2 medium | 504 |
| Winter squash | ½ cup | 473 |

## The Foods Recommended by Ann Wigmore

Ann Wigmore devised a diet consisting primarily of raw, unadulterated foods. "Living foods" are a direct way to revitalize the body and supply the energy necessary for healing. People came to her mansion in Boston from all over the world to heal themselves of all sorts of intractable diseases, including cancer. The living foods scene has expanded considerably since then, so I will try to resurrect the original concept in all its simplicity.

Wigmore's healing diet consisted of:

- **Uncooked fruits and vegetables**

- **Sprouted greens** from alfalfa, sunflower, and other seeds for enzymes and phytosterols

- **Sprouted nut and sunflower seed cheeses,** more potent as cancer fighters than carrot juice [52]

- **Sprouted seed and nut milks**, especially sesame, almond, and sunflower, major sources of phytosterols and essential fatty acids

- **Wheatgrass juice** and other dark green juice

- **Fermented foods** such as four-day sauerkraut to aid digestion and heal leaky gut

- **Rejuvelac,** a drink made from fermented wheat, that supplies *Lactobacilli, Saccharomyces,* and *Aspergillus oryzae*

- **Watermelon or raw applesauce** breakfasts for flushing the kidneys

- **Complete meal soups made from raw vegetables**

- **Grain crisps,** uncooked sprouted grain breads ("Essene" bread) made in a food dryer

- **Other valuable foods** such as parsley, prunes, alfalfa, avocado, dates and figs, Jerusalem artichokes, apples, carob, dulse, kelp, and garden weeds

- **Foods dried in season at very low temperatures** (under 105°) in a food dryer to retain most of their nutritional value

## Mental and Spiritual Effects of a High Energy Diet

- A high energy diet can bestow a natural high—joy, charisma, increased energy, and more loving responses to others. This natural high supplies a forward momentum which speeds healing.

- Living foods have a calming effect on the emotions, making it easier to cope with stress, and improving the quality of sleep.

- A living foods diet alleviates depression, minimizing the obsessive thoughts that plague many illnesses.

- High energy food breaks down emotional armoring, opening a way for natural release and integration of repressed emotion.

- Living foods revive a will which has been weakened by drugs and highly processed food. This includes the will to survive and the will to choose the best foods rather than passively taking a chance with whatever comes our way.

• Intuition grows stronger, improving our ability to listen to the body telling us what it needs. A body free of addictions can be trusted.

• Living foods provide a connection with the life force, an energy that cannot be measured in food tables. This energy comes directly from the sun through the process of photosynthesis.

• This is a friendly way to eat. No animals are killed.

## Organically Grown Live Foods

• Are free of the addictive chemicals added to fast foods and processed foods.

• Do not need enhancement with salt because they do not lose their flavor through cooking.

• Contain no trans fatty acids from hydrogenated oils and margarine. These acids interfere with uptake of the omega-3 oils necessary for countering inflammation.

• Provide high fiber for prevention of colon cancer and restoration of bowel function.

• Contain much higher levels of natural minerals.

• Are more alkaline and do not supply the acid environment necessary for mucus production. Lower production of mucus allows clearing of lymph and liver for freer removal of toxins.

• Are easier on the digestive system and liver. Alkaline foods carry their own enzymes and fiber and do not cause problems with acid indigestion or constipation.

- Are rejuvenating.

## Why Eat Sprouts?

Sprouts contain more enzymes, minerals, amino acids, and vitamins than other vegetables.

- Beans, grains, and seeds become more digestible when sprouted.

- Minerals become more bioavailable.

- Sprouts can be grown inexpensively in your kitchen.

# Juicing and Juice Feasting For Energy

The live juice healing program developed by Dr. Max Gerson over seventy years ago is a prototype program for healing with food. Albert Schweitzer, after being healed of tuberculosis by using Dr. Gerson's methods, considered Gerson a medical genius because of his understanding of the relationship of food to illness. The number of people who have recovered from cancer and other serious illness (including Lyme disease) through this program is astonishing. Though this regimen is very demanding, many people choose it because of the success rate. They usually require assistance from others, mainly to help with hourly juice-making (see appendix).

In the cancerous body a combination of factors is at work. Cancer cells grow in conditions of low oxygen and fermentation of sugars—this slowly poisons the entire organism; the electrical activity in the vital organs diminishes and the liver is weakened to the point where it cannot defend the body against malignancy or other onslaught. A state of low oxygen and fermentation of sugars is also present in many chronic diseases. Gerson believed that working with such conditions requires three basic approaches:

1. Detoxify the body by neutralizing acidity with alkaline juices.

2. Fortify the body with minerals from the potassium group.

3. Provide a constant supply of enzymes to support the body until it is able to support itself.

Restoration of the proper ratio of potassium requires restriction of salt and sodium in foods, as salt cancels out potassium. The Gerson program requires intake of eight ounces of fresh juice thirteen times a day, combined with potassium supplementation to restore potassium levels and to neutralize and force excretion of salt. Of the juices, carrot is the most frequently used.

## Creating a Juicing Lifestyle

Though most people would probably not be able to devote themselves 100% to juicing, it is possible to incorporate various levels of juicing into a program of health restoration. Juicing is not a cure all, though if one followed a Gerson-type program it could be. Juicing simply gives your body support and energy for the fight.

Why juicing instead of water fasting? Many detoxification experts say we are so loaded with toxins these days that rapid detoxification can lead to severe problems if toxins are so rapidly excreted that they go back into circulation. Juicing offers a way to manage this process in a gradual and sensible way. I believe the drinking of large quantities of juice to be more productive, for it provides colossal amounts of nutrition and it does not shock the body. Periodic juice feasting is safe. Many studies indicate that even long water-fasts do not lead to malnutrition or other damage.[53]

## Three Levels of Juicing

**Juicing Level 1: Awakened Curiosity.** Drink at least a quart of mostly green juice every day, adding, if desired, a few super food supplements such as spirulina, herbal tinctures, or liquid minerals. This will assure adequate nutrition, attention to the liver, a certain amount of detoxification, and energy to get started in the morning. This practice will form a strong foundation for resisting or even keeping ahead of Lyme.

**Juicing Level 2: Going for the Wisdom.** This would qualify as the early stages of "juice feasting." Here you would drink at least 2 quarts of juice a day, with an 80% raw diet free of allergenic, addictive, or otherwise offending foods. From this you may expect to feel increased motivation, marked increases in energy, more creative thinking, inspiration, and discipline for carrying through with protocols. Cellular aliveness and lymph clearing increase early and noticeably.

**Juicing Level 3: Riding the Wave.** Juice-feasting involves drinking three or four quarts of fresh, mostly green juice a day. You get the benefits of fasting without the risks, while building up and replenishing the body's store of essential nutrients. What can you expect from this? Usually it brings high, almost ecstatic energy that radiates out to the world. If you can do this long enough, you could expect dramatic healing of many of the conditions caused by modern lifestyles. I have to admit that this is not easy to do. However, it is a worthy goal to aim for if you can refrain from criticizing yourself if you slip up and go off your routine. "Feasting" means to eat heartily with delight. One can find online juice feasters who claim to drink four quarts a day for up to 100 days. Even just a day or two of this will pleasantly energize your system.

# Level 1 And 2: Adopting a Juicing Lifestyle

As the number one remedial food therapy, energizer and alkalizer of the body, juices incorporate easily into daily life and should be done over the longer term (like forever). There are a few basic ground rules:

**Make juice first thing in the morning** before you talk yourself out of it or get involved in other things.

**Drink your fresh juice on an empty stomach** in order to avoid digestive problems.

**Avoid all canned or frozen juices.** Commercial fruit juices are big blasts of sugar. They are usually not organically grown and contain virtually no enzymes.

**Juices should be used fresh from the juicer** before they have a chance to oxidize. They should be stored in the refrigerator immediately, to be used the same day. However, they will keep a little longer if no air gets to them (as in a vacuum seal).

**Juice anything and everything.** Often when people begin a healing journey, they will say they don't like kale, or spinach, or any number of things. It is possible to create combinations which include small amounts of foods you don't like if you add small amounts of them to a large enough quantity of other juices to hide the taste. Experiment! Be sure of getting a variety: "forage around" in your natural food store or organic farmers' market. Try vegetables you have never tried. Get creative with your juicing and it will never get boring.

**It is OK to mix fruit and vegetable juices together.** Ordinarily combining fruits and vegetables would be considered poor food combining. However, most of the digestive work is accomplished in the breaking down process of juicing.

**Juice for as long or as little as you like.** You can incorporate one or more short juice feasts into your lifestyle. Decide how many days of the year to do this, and make time for this. Some prefer to have nothing but juice one day a week, some for a few days a month or longer. Proceed gently rather than forcing an agenda you might not be ready for.

**Get a juicer that will get the most out of your greens.** The best juicer is the very expensive Norwalk ($2,500 range), followed by Greenstar ($300-$400 range) or other twin-gear juicer. Cheap juicers and other spin-type juicers will not produce good enough juice for long-term healing. The spinning action oxidizes the juices quickly, reducing their effectiveness.

# Level 3 Juice Feasting

Juice feasting undoes some of the damage brought on by years of destructive creature-comfort foods and negative attitudes to life that have dampened the fire within and led to premature decay of the physical body.

- It creates an alkaline condition in the body which spirochetes cannot tolerate.

- The body begins to consume anything it does not need, such as excess fat, toxins, and metabolic wastes that clog the system. It helps to decongest the lymph, the blood flow and the thinking processes.

- It activates the liver.

- It repairs the digestive system and rebuilds other organs. This frees the system of irritating, undigested debris that contributes to toxic thoughts (via the leaky gut route). Good digestion can eliminate depressive states, improve mood, and reduce irritability. Life looks good!

- Cravings and addictions, as well as allergies, go away. They will stay gone as long as you do not revert to the old habits after the feast is over.

- Juice feasting is rejuvenating: people who juice-feast up to a couple weeks or more can look years younger. Slowing of the aging process is an obvious sign that cell repair is happening.

- It rebuilds the immune system, replenishing the supply of glutathione.

- It can reduce inflammation and pain.

- It brings oxygen to all cells of the body, relieving chronic fatigue and fibromyalgia.

- Cholesterol and blood pressure levels go down.

- Tension and insomnia improve or disappear.

- It offers freedom from those long lists of supplements.

- It is delicious: it is hard to get tired of fresh juices. There is no food that the body welcomes more. The energy it brings to the cells is real and tangible.

## Feasting Is About Inner Abundance and Whole-Hearted Generosity to Self

Juice feasting can deliver a natural high, heightening the mental drive to stay committed, hopeful, and positive. The improved energy, clarity, and peacefulness strengthen the will, making it considerably easier to carry out other healing activities willingly and with intention.

The strengthened power of will carries over into the broader areas of life, making it easier to succeed at other ventures as well. Juice-feasting brings with it a vision of abundance, health, and harmony that bestows on you the power to create. You feel less imprisoned by the exterior world and its demanding ways. Juice feasting is a way to heed and nurture wholeness of body and mind. It is quality time spent with your own being. Temporarily removing the stimulus of food makes room for the mind to engage in deeper healing in a natural state of meditation. This deeper state of mind approaches the ecstatic, energetic love-brain where true self-healing can occur.

## Feasting Should Be Done in an Environment Conducive To Healing

It is desirable to be in a living situation free of stress, emotional upset or physical strain. It is particularly important to avoid high-stress people who need a lot of stimulation and attention. Rest and peaceful surroundings are best. Be around people who support you in what you are doing and can perhaps join you in feasting.

# Take Care of Your Body

Maintain exercise in moderation. Many people report that they are able to perform remarkable physical feats on juice. But a person who is sick may need to preserve the new-found energy and build up a hoard of energy in the body. If possible, get massages, steam baths, and anything else that keeps the system moving. As you move into a more spiritual state, devote more time to spiritual practices such as *pranayama*, meditation and qigong.

# Avoid Temptation

Do not tantalize yourself by watching junk food commercials on television or putting yourself in places where cooking aromas fill the air. Find other juice feasters online and get encouragement from their stories.

# Starting a Juice Feast

It is advisable to consult with a (naturopathic) doctor knowledgeable about your condition to determine whether juicing is feasible for you. It is important to have a physician who will not undermine your efforts: he or she should ideally practice juicing in their own life or at least have enough experience of it to understand how it works.

# Withdrawing From Addictions

Addictions to alcohol, nicotine, caffeine, or sugar should be reduced slowly. Some people prefer to do this over a few weeks, and some prefer to use the cold turkey method and endure the sudden withdrawal. Do not be tempted to accommodate an addiction, even just a little, since eating the food which you crave will start the craving cycle all over. Withdrawal from addictions means complete withdrawal. Eating only fresh fruits and vegetables is a good way to start a withdrawal (no sugar, meat, eggs, or dairy during withdrawal).

## Traditional Indications to Stop or Modify Any Healing Routine

- **Extreme discomfort is a sign to discontinue any extreme dietary change.**

- Persistent arrhythmias or unstable angina can be caused by acidity and sodium/potassium imbalances. If extra potassium does not correct this, stop what you are doing until the pre-existing condition is remedied.[54]

- Kidney or gallstone attacks. Proceed slowly if you have gallbladder problems in order to forestall gallbladder attacks. If an attack does happen, stop right away and do whatever you usually do when this happens. Be sure to drink plenty of water.

- Acute ulcerative condition of the gastro-duodenal tract (rare) calls for a gradual healing. Repeated, careful, short periods of juicing will heal this condition.

- Hypoglycemic persons need to be cautious that they do not become too disrupted. A short juice feast may be more advisable than a long one. You need to determine whether certain juices are too sweet for the present condition of the body.

## End Your Juice Feasting When Your Body Tells You To

Stick with the juices until you feel you have juiced long enough. Prematurely adding solid food to your diet can tempt you to end your feast too soon. You have not been starving yourself, but rather stoking yourself with high nutrition.

Get off the juice feast gradually. Do not celebrate the end of your feast with hog-wild food choices. Return to regular eating with sensible, easy-to-digest foods. No pizza or burritos for a while!

# Juices

**Juicers:** If you do not have a good juicer, please note that it is always better to use a cheap juicer than none at all.

**Greens** are the supreme food of this planet, the best detoxifiers and energizers. George Washington Carver maintained that plants such as sheep sorrel, peppergrass, wild chicory, and dandelions, which grow in nature, are far superior to those devitalized by cultivation. The renowned French herbal healer, Maurice Mességué felt that by using herbs indiscriminately on a daily basis in juices and teas, he could incorporate into his body the qualities of each herb, thus becoming those qualities. He believed the drinking of one or two green teas such as nettle or red clover could dramatically affect an illness. Some dark green leafy vegetables to juice are:

Amaranth

Beet greens

Bok choi and other Asian greens

Chard

Cilantro

Endive

Lamb's quarter

Parsley

Romaine

Spinach

Wheatgrass

Wild greens such as chickweed, dandelion, kudzu, lamb's quarter, purslane, and sorrel

**Cruciferous vegetables** supply the sulfide that helps prevent clogging of blood vessels. Best known as a source of sulfur (sulfurothane) are broccoli and broccoli sprouts. Small quantities of broccoli sprouts may be as nutritive as large quantities of mature plants. Broccoli stems not used in cooking may be juiced along with other juices. Other cruciferous vegetables to consider adding to the diet are

> Brussels sprouts
>
> Cabbage
>
> Cauliflower
>
> Horseradish
>
> Kohlrabi
>
> Mustard greens
>
> Red, white or black radish
>
> Rutabaga
>
> Turnip greens
>
> Watercress
>
> Mustard greens

# Other Potent Juices

**Beets:** start with small amounts and work up to remedial doses slowly.

**Black radish:** add a small piece to your juice. Beets and black radish juices are so potent that they should be considered medicine and used judiciously. Start with a wineglass-sized portion of beet juice and less than an ounce of black radish juice to start the bile juices moving again.

**Carrot juice** is the mainstay of the Gerson program. Turning yellow from drinking too much carrot juice is harmless unless you drink huge quantities over several years. The yellow is due to a factor in carrots, not to an overworked liver. Elevated levels of beta-carotene do not lead to vitamin A toxicity. There are those who would tell you not to drink carrot juice because it is so sweet. The heavy use of carrot juice in the Gerson program to fight cancer would suggest that this is not harmful. Carrot goes well with other vegetables and is a good base for almost anything. It can make green vegetable juices more palatable.

**Lemons and limes** (fresh) make strong-tasting green juices more palatable. Juice half a lime or more with any creative mixture you might find hard to drink. Strong juices may also be thinned by adding fresh cucumber, zucchini, or other watery juice.

**Fresh burdock root:** add a small stick or two to other juices for added medicinal power. Burdock activates the liver and kidneys. It is easy to juice and it has a pleasant taste. Start with one small root and build up to an amount that is tolerable for you. The appropriate amount may vary from person to person, depending on the amount of cleansing it causes. You can find fresh burdock root in most oriental stores or natural food stores in season. Burdock tincture may be added to juice if the fresh root is not available.

**Juice Popsicles.** A quantity of some of the more medicinal juices may be frozen in ice cube trays and kept in the freezer. Add a cube or two to juices or smoothies at any time. Burdock and wheatgrass juice work well this way. Other likely candidates for this are black radish juice, beet juice, and juices from fresh medicinal herbs such as milk thistle, dandelion, and chickweed.

**Fruit.** Many people like to add a lot of fruit to juices and smoothies. Too much fruit adds too much fructose to the diet. It is best to stick with low-fructose fruits on a healing diet. Fruits lowest in fructose are limes, lemons, cranberries, raspberries, strawberries, and blackberries. Fruits such as watermelons, pears, raisins, dates and dried fruit, seedless grapes, and mangoes are highest in fructose.

| Fruit[55] | Serving Size | Gms of Fructose |
|---|---|---|
| Limes | 1 medium | 0 |
| Lemons | 1 medium | 0.6 |
| Cranberries | 1 cup | 0.7 |
| Prune | 1 medium | 1.2 |
| Date (Deglet Noor) | 1 medium | 2.6 |
| Cantaloupe | 1/8 of med. melon | 2.8 |
| Raspberries | 1 cup | 3.0 |
| Kiwifruit | 1 medium | 3.4 |
| Blackberries | 1 cup | 3.5 |
| Cherries, sweet | 10 | 3.8 |
| Strawberries | 1 cup | 3.8 |
| Cherries, sour | 1 cup | 4.0 |
| Pineapple | 1 slice (3.5" x .75") | 4.0 |
| Grapefruit, pink or red | 1/2 medium | 4.3 |
| Boysenberries | 1 cup | 4.6 |
| Tangerine/ mandarin orange | 1 medium | 4.8 |
| Nectarine | 1 medium | 5.4 |

| | | |
|---|---|---|
| Peach | 1 medium | 5.9 |
| Orange (navel) | 1 medium | 6.1 |
| Papaya | 1/2 medium | 6.3 |
| Honeydew | 1/8 of med. melon | 6.7 |
| Banana | 1 medium | 7.1 |
| Blueberries | 1 cup | 7.4 |
| Date (Medjool) | 1 medium | 7.7 |
| Apple (composite) | 1 medium | 9.5 |
| Watermelon | 1/16 med. melon | 11.3 |
| Pear | 1 medium | 11.8 |
| Raisins | 1/4 cup | 12.3 |
| Grapes, seedless | 1 cup | 12.4 |
| Mango | 1/2 medium | 16.2 |
| Apricots, dried | 1 cup | 16.4 |
| Figs, dried | 1 cup | 23.0 |

# Juice Combinations

There is no great mystery to juice combinations. Almost anything can go into a juice or smoothie. Adding a little lime or lemon juice usually makes anything taste good. Fresh pineapple rescues any combination, but is high in sugar content. I encourage people to experiment and invent their own favorite mixes.

A good basic juice consists of greens and carrots. Cucumber or zucchini, for example, may be added to this for variety. Apple is popular in juices, but again, pay attention to the sugar content. Keep fruit combinations to a minimum and stick with the low-sugar fruits, if necessary.

I include the following two juice combinations to illustrate how great combinations can happen spontaneously from vegetables you might have around:

## Subterranean Putzfrau Earth Juice

This powerful juice cleanser hits all the avenues of detoxification at once. It brings about a dramatic output of bile and increases urination. If you take a glass of this first thing in the morning every day for a week, you will find your liver working better, your mood improving, and your overall sense of wellbeing returning.

¼ or less of 1 medium black radish (for bowel and lymphatic system)

½ medium sized beet (for liver)

1 -8" piece of burdock root (for liver and kidney)

1 clove garlic (for everything)

¾" piece of ginger root (for digestion)

6 or more carrots (for the liver and to add flavor)

Greens as desired

## Carrot Alexander

10 carrots

2 stalks celery

Fresh mint to taste

# Green Smoothies

Green smoothies can be an alternative or a complement to juicing. Juicing leaves pulp, whereas smoothies use the whole plant, including all the phytosterols in the fiber. Pulp left over from juicing or making seed milks may be added to smoothies. When making smoothies, it is best to emphasize greens over fruit because of sugar content.

Doing a green smoothie feast rather than a juice feast is also a great tool for healing. It gives you the added benefit of feeling like you are taking in solid food.

## Benefits of Making Smoothies with Greens

- The greens are more easily broken down and digested; nutrients are better absorbed.

- This is the best fast food on the planet.

- Since you use the whole food, there is no waste (and no guilt feelings).

- The fibers in the greens are a major source of roughage.

- Food fibers contain the phytosterols.

- Food fibers are very healing for leaky gut.

- Smoothies allow you to incorporate some of the less tasty greens into the diet.

- Smoothies will keep for up to 3 days in the refrigerator (though it is better to drink them fresh). This allows you to make the day's supply ahead of time.

- Smoothie recipes are not complex: almost anything can find its way into a smoothie and still taste good.

**Equipment**: the best blenders for the job are **Blendtec or Vitamix** ($400 and $500 respectively). But any decent blender will do if the consistency of the smoothie is not a consideration, i.e. if you don't mind your smoothie being a little gloppy.

## Basic Procedure for Making Smoothies

1. Blend fruits first. Use a ratio of 30% fruits to 70% greens.

2. Cover ingredients with water or fresh juice.

3. Blend until smooth, but not hot. If your blender makes things hot, add ice cubes.

4. Drink right away or store in refrigerator for up to three days. Smoothies keep longer than juices, so make enough for the whole day and possibly for the next morning.

## Ingredients

* Any leafy greens, though it is best to limit the quantities of greens which have a high content of oxalic acid such as spinach, chard, amaranth leaves, and sorrel. Baby spinach does not contain as much oxalic acid as fully grown spinach.

* Use freely: kale, romaine, watercress, mustard greens, cabbage, turnip greens, carrot tops, and broccoli. Kale and collard leaves should be stripped from the coarse stalk.

* If you need to be careful about fructose, use low-sugar fruits.

* If you want a creamy smoothie, add some avocado or banana.

## Juices and Smoothies as Vehicles for Other Concentrated Foods

* Powdered Chinese herbs

* Aloe vera powder

- Biotin powder for liver and brain
- Omega-3 fish oils if camouflaged by lemon juice
- Flax oil
- Almond, sunflower, or sesame mush left over from making seed milks
- Ground up nuts
- Kelp powder, dulse or other soft seaweed
- Lemon juice, blended with chopped peel; lime juice
- MSM powder
- Spirulina, chlorella, barley green; green powder concentrates
- Bee pollen, royal jelly
- Frozen popsicles: wheatgrass, burdock, beet juice
- One or more cloves of fresh garlic
- Piece of fresh ginger root; powdered or minced ginger
- Dash of capsicum for extra cleansing power
- Herbal tinctures or teas; green tea
- Buffered vitamin C powder
- Supplements: powdered or liquid magnesium, inositol; liquid iodine supplement
- Protein powders such as pumpkin seed or hemp seed. Whey protein isolate is broken down by fruit juices, so it should be used alone.
- Rejuvelac
- Lecithin powder or granules
- Magnesium powder or other mineral powders

- Liquid iodine drops

- Powdered kelp or other seaweed

## Monster Mash Limonene Cadillac Smoothie (Second Generation Whole Lemon Drink)

This is an example of a smoothie taken to extremes. You may add as many superfoods to a smoothie as you can tolerate. Since I am not known to be a kitchen goddess, I like to put as much nutrition into the things I do make. So I have expanded on the basic formula for whole lemon drink and turned it into a powerhouse smoothie for breakfast. These ingredients may vary from day to day:

½ of a lemon, including rind

Juice of 2 limes or 1 apple

Cranberries or other berries in moderation

Entire bunch of parsley, collards, kale, or other greens

1 small beet or piece of a beet

1-4 cloves of garlic (start with one)


Add various supplements such as:

1 or more ounces of fish oil (lemon conceals the taste)

¼ tsp. or more of high BTU cayenne (hot)

1 tsp. of pureed ginger

Magnesium powder or liquid magnesium chloride

Iodine drops (work up gradually to an appropriate dose)

Leftover mush from making seed milks

8-16 ounces of water or more

Mix these ingredients in Vitamix until they are liquefied. If this mixture is hard to drink, use smaller portions of difficult parts such as the lemon peel, garlic, or cayenne. It is possible to make this quite delicious by tailoring the ingredients to taste.

## Personal Comment

Which is better, juices or smoothies? After doing just green smoothies for the past year and then recently going back to good old carrot juice, I have to say that the smoothies do not give me the energy blast that carrot juice does. This energy has great calmative benefits as well. This is such a good feeling that I always look forward to my next batch of juice.

I can't compare the nutritional qualities of juices versus smoothies because I have no way to measure that. The bottom line here is that when you get tired of juice you can go to smoothies, and when you get tired of smoothies you can go to juices. That makes it much easier to stay powerfully and consistently connected to the fresh, raw, vegetable world.

I do not know whether other people have a problem with the high calcium content of carrot juice. I find it necessary to add some magnesium powder to balance it and to keep me from getting leg cramps.

# EIGHT

# A Little Help from Supplements

Keeping the immune system healthy and mobilizing it against disease would depend more on giving the body systemic support than on deploying tailored magic immunotherapeutics. Proven immunomodulators such as mushroom extracts take on significant relevance. Fish oils, vitamin C, glutathione, and other antioxidants, as well as numerous plant extracts can further enhance immune cell functionality . . . As heroic efforts to tailor technological immune therapies go forward, the best immune intervention tools continue to be lifestyle modification, vitamins, minerals, orthomolecules, and selected nontoxic phytotherapies.

Paris Kidd [56]

**Support:** It is an art to know when to search out and receive outside help.

Taking supplements is another discipline to acquire, and most people find it hard, for various reasons, to swallow a handful of pills every day. I list here a few top supplements for maintenance. Supplements and herbs for active disease or flare-ups have been well documented by others (Buhner, et al). Once it becomes apparent that one is dealing with a chronic situation, the supplements below can be instrumental in helping you maintain a degree of wellness and function.

This list of supplements could get quite a bit longer if specific needs for flare-ups or co-infections were taken into consideration. Those listed here are candidates for long-term use. It has taken me a long time to decide which are truly worth taking, so I hope this list will prove useful for others. While I would prefer to get it all through foods, adding a few supplements could just provide a good one-two punch to your self-healing efforts.

## Vitamin B12

B12 is an essential partner in immune function, as it is a crucial link in the methylation cycle. It helps maintain myelin in the brain and plays a part in the formation of red blood cells. Signs of deficiency are anemia (tiredness, weakness), depression, dizziness, poor balance, tinnitus, memory problems, poor coordination, panic attacks, multiple sclerosis, and neuropathies. Serious B12 deficiency manifests in dementia and neurological damage so serious that it can be mistaken for Alzheimer's. Persons suffering from autoimmune illnesses are prone to B12 deficiencies.

The preferred form of B12 is methylcobalamin, more expensive than the readily available cyanocobalamin form. B12 is best taken sublingually or by self-administered shots. It is a good idea to take a complete B-complex along with this in order to maintain a proper ratio of B vitamins. Food sources of B12 are eggs, meat and dairy products. Spirulina contains small amounts of B12.

## Vitamin D3

Lack of vitamin D3 is now thought to be a major player in the pathology of many serious health conditions. It plays a role in preventing cancer, in stimulating the immune system and regulating inflammation. Deficiency may be determined by a blood test. Though it is vital to have adequate levels of D3, too much D3 can lead to the dangerous condition of hypercalcemia, or too much calcium in the blood. Therefore, a vitamin D supplement with added Vitamin K2 is the preferred form for preventing this.

## Best sources of D3 are:

- The sun. A half hour exposure to the sun twice a week is considered adequate.

- Best food source: 1 tablespoon of cod liver oil provides 1,360 IU of Vitamin D, a safe daily dosage.

## Magnesium

*Borrelia* spirochetes usurp magnesium from the body. Many of the familiar symptoms of Lyme look like the symptoms of magnesium deficiency: muscle and joint problems, muscle cramps, twitching and tics, tremors, depression, insomnia, short-term memory problems, cognitive difficulties, heart palpitations, inflammation, reduced immune function,[57] food cravings of all sorts, mood problems, bowel inflammation, chronic fatigue and fibromyalgia, hyperactivity, premenstrual syndrome, restless leg syndrome, metabolic syndrome, and shortness of breath.

Magnesium is necessary for maintaining proper calcium balance in the body. Magnesium deficiency may account in part for recurrences of Lyme in spite of antibiotic therapy. Magnesium is, therefore, considered an immune stimulator.[58]

Of the supplements, magnesium glycinate is believed to be free of the laxative effect other forms of magnesium have. Magnesium supplements are better absorbed when taken with food. It is probably possible to obtain enough magnesium from proper foods. The best food sources of magnesium are almonds and other nuts, blackstrap molasses, wheat bran, wheat germ and green leafy vegetables.

Magnesium oil (liquid magnesium chloride) can provide topical relief from muscle spasms: when applied directly to the skin it will usually stop the spasms. Magnesium chloride is also available in powder form for use in foot soaks and magnesium baths.

# LDN (Low Dose Naltrexone)

LDN is not truly a natural supplement, and it is available only by prescription. Naltrexone was originally used in 50 mg doses in the treatment of heroin addicts to block opioid receptors in the brain and other body cells, including those of the immune system. In 1985 Dr. Bernard Bihari discovered that much smaller doses, taken at bedtime, enhance the immune system of persons with HIV by preventing deterioration in CD4 helper T cells. It was later discovered that low dose naltrexone could help many people with autoimmune diseases or cancer keep their disease under control.

Research is showing that the body's own secretions of endorphins, its internal opioids, are necessary for the immune system. They play a part in the formation, differentiation, and role of immune cells. These benefits occur if the opioid receptors are blocked between 2 a.m. and 4 a.m. in the morning, when an increase in endorphin and enkephalin production occurs. This causes an increase in natural killer (NK) cells and other immune defenses. Since cancer and autoimmune diseases are associated with a deficiency of endorphins, stimulating production of endorphins with LDN can vitalize the immune system. At the very least, LDN can improve quality of life with no side effects.[59]

Though Lyme disease is not mentioned in the literature, the list of autoimmune diseases which have been shown to benefit from LDN suggests that Lyme would also benefit. Many doctors are now aware of LDN and prescribe it regularly for:

- Chronic fatigue syndrome

- HIV/AIDS

- Multiple sclerosis

- Psoriasis

- Hepatitis C

- Rheumatoid arthritis

- Systemic lupus

The recommended dosage is 3 to 4.5 mg at bedtime. Be sure you do not get the slow-release LDN. When you first start taking LDN you will probably find yourself more inclined to wakefulness at night. However, this will eventually wear off and sleep will return to normal. A nice side-effect of LDN is its remarkable effect on dreams—they become much more powerful and colorful.

## Cautionary Warnings

1.  People using narcotic medication or codeine-containing medication should get these drugs completely out of their system before taking LDN. This may take up to two weeks of gradual withdrawal.

2.  Persons taking thyroid hormone replacement for Hashimoto's thyroiditis with hypothyroidism need to start LDN at the lowest range (1.5mg for an adult). Since LDN may improve autoimmune disorders, thyroid medication dose may need to be reduced in accordance with that.

3.  LDN may interfere with immunosuppressive medication.

## Vitamin C

Vitamin C is required for the production of glutathione. But it also has another use which I have found helpful for neurotoxin symptoms (the "head full of mush" syndrome). A vitamin C flush taken first thing in the morning usually reduces the discomfort from flare-ups of brain fog and Herxheimer reactions. Another notice-able effect of a vitamin C flush is a dramatic increase in energy, always a welcome event.

Vitamin C flushes, as described on the Perque website,[60] may be done over time, once a week or as needed. The stated purpose of the vitamin C flush is to determine vitamin C deficiency. It in-volves taking 3 g (1 level tsp.) of buffered vitamin C powder every 15 minutes until you reach a large enough dose to begin having watery stools. 75% of that amount would then be what you would take for a daily dose.

| Number Of Level Tsps. (1 Tsp. =3 G) | Total Ascorbate Consumed | Approximate Daily (75%) Therapeutic Dose (Level Tsps.) |
|---|---|---|
| 3 | 9 | 7 |
| 5 | 15 | 12 |
| 12.5 | 37.5 | 19 |
| 45 | 135 | 101 |

A general daily dose of vitamin C would be 3-6 g. The benefits of vitamin C may be summarized as follows:

- Improves function of the immune system and enhances glutathione production.

- Neutralizes and removes toxins.

- Reduces heavy metal toxicity.

- Repairs and forms collagen.

- Helps joint function.

- Produces energy.

- Is an antioxidant.

# Adaptogens

Adaptogens remedy stress, a dominant factor in chronic disease. Though adaptogens are popularly thought of as stimulating, they do not have the same physiological effects as chemical stimulants. They are commonly used for immune restoration, nerve system repair, and possible hormone regulation. Listed here are several of the most popular adaptogens, although many others could be helpful as well. They have been shown to:

- Support the adrenals in coping with stress.

- Help the body generate more energy, both physical and mental.

- Aid in the elimination of toxins.

- Improve the way the body uses oxygen.

- Reduce fatigue.

## Some adaptogenic herbs are:

- Eleuthero

- Schizandra

- Reishi mushrooms

- Ashwaganda

- Gotu kola

- Wild oats

- Astragalus or *huang chi*

- *Fo-ti* or *ho shou wu*

- Burdock

- Suma

Three adaptogens are often mentioned in discussions of Lyme:

**Rhodiola rosea** was the herb of choice for the ancient Vikings when they needed strength for their fighting and pillaging excursions. It helped them cope with a cold climate and a stressful life. Rhodiola should be taken in the morning, starting with a small dose (100 mg) and building up slowly over time. If it makes you jittery after taking it for a while, it is best to stop. Though rhodiola has been found to relieve depression,[61] it should not be taken by people who are bipolar or manic.

**Reishi mushrooms** (*Ganoderma*) can assist in recovery from a flare up or crash. It seems to be able to re-engage the immune system. In China these mushrooms were thought to confer immortality on the eater. The *Nei Pien* of Po Hung describes the mushrooms:

> They may resemble buildings, palanquins and horses, dragons and tigers, human beings, or flying birds. They may be any of the five colors . . . When dried in the shade, powdered, and taken by the inch-square spoonful, they produce geniehood. Those of the intermediate class confer several thousands of years and those of the lowest type a thousand years of life.[62]

**Resveratrol from Japanese Knotweed** (*Polygonum cuspidatum*). Japanese knotweed is a core herb of the Buhner protocol for Lyme. While it has all the properties of most adaptogens, it is particularly useful for Lyme arthritis and for minimizing Herxheimer reactions. Buhner recommends using whole herb supplements rather than just resveratrol supplements because other constituents of the plant are powerfully synergistic. He recommends beginning with 1 tablet per day for one week, adding another tablet per day the second week, and so on. When you reach the maximum dose, stay on it for at least 60 days, and then gradually lower it if symptoms have improved. Japanese Knotweed grows wild in a number of places, so an enterprising person could gather their own to use in teas or to roll into capsules. Roots should be dug in the fall from first year plants. This plant is considered a seriously noxious weed. All sorts of attacks on it seem to fail. If you find a patch of it, be sure it has not been poisoned.

## Systemic Enzymes

**Caution:** Systemic enzymes, including lumbrokinase and nattokinase, should not be used by anyone who is hemophiliac or using prescription blood thinners, as this combination may thin the blood too much.

Elevated fibrinogen is found in persons with fibromyalgia, mycoplasma, chronic pain, migraine, Lyme disease and babesia. Fibrin provides a hiding place where microbial pathogens can avoid detection by the immune system.

Systemic enzyme formulas will scavenge anything that should not be in your body such as scar tissue and fibrin deposited in organs and blood vessels. They help prevent strokes and heart attacks caused by blood clots and enable white blood cells to combat infection.

Enzymes work against "Lyme biofilm" which is responsible for the persistence of chronic Lyme and its co-infections. The biofilm is a protective film that envelops microbes and prevents the immune system from recognizing them. The biofilm also provides nutrition for the microbes. It is hypothesized that the biofilms in neurological Lyme disease are built from the myelin which protects the nerves. This causes the immune system to attack the central nervous system as it tries to break through the biofilm to get to the infection. When biofilms are removed the immune system is more able to destroy the microbes.

Peta Cohen, M.S., R.D. explains biofilms:

Bacteria build biofilms by first aggregating together, and then rapidly weaving this protective web or matrix around them. They build a polymeric matrix. It's a sticky, gluey, mucus-y goop and it's got fibrin in it to give it an intact structure. The bacteria recruit fibrinogen to create fibrin as part of that matrix. At that point they can shed their outer membrane, which has the proteins that serve as antigens and as a target of the missile of the immune system. They're very protected. They're very crafty in creating a way to survive and procreate and hide from the immune system.[63]

Cohen uses a combination of things to treat autism. He believes this therapy can also treat Lyme, lupus, and MS. His protocol consists of:

- The enzymes nattokinase and lumbrokinase

- EDTA

- Antimicrobials such as grapefruit seed extract, or GSE; echinacea, goldenseal, gentian, tea tree oil, oregano oil, neem

- Binders such as citrus pectin and aluminum free sodium bicarbonate

- Buffering agents (i.e. vitamin C)

Enzymes should be taken on an empty stomach with plenty of water first thing in the morning and last thing at night. Recommended enzymes are Wobenzym.

**Lumbrokinase, Nattokinase.** The enzymes lumbrokinase and nattokinase are thought to be more effective at removing the bacterial biofilms that make treatment of Lyme so difficult. Lumbrokinase is derived from earthworms and is used in China to treat nerve diseases, dissolve blood clots and vein thrombosis, protect against heart disease and strokes, and lower fibrinogen levels in cancer patients.

Nattokinase has similar properties, though it may be less effective than the earthworm formula. It has been used for 1,000 years in Japan. It is extracted from a traditional Japanese food called "natto," a fermented soybean product.

"Lyme fog" is partially caused by a formation of amyloid deposits in the brain which prevent the cells from functioning properly. Researchers report that nattokinase (not trypsin or plasmin) can cut into the amyloid and facilitate its removal.

Nattokinase can

- Clear the brain of biofilms as well as amyloid proteins.

- Quickly clear out organisms hiding in blood platelets in difficult cases of Lyme.

- Stabilize blood pressure and fortify veins and arteries against high blood pressure and hypertension.

- Stop the hypercoagulation linked to many heart problems, fibromyalgia, and chronic fatigue syndrome.

**Caution:** Since nattokinase is an anti-coagulant, it must be used with care. Cuts need to be promptly cared for if one is using anti-coagulants.

## Milk Thistle Seed

Milk-thistle (*Silybum marianum*) is the go-to herb for the liver. It is the source of silymarin, which:

- Helps preserve glutathione levels and enhance detoxification in the liver. It can increase glutathione levels by up to 35%. Silymarin is a more potent antioxidant than both vitamins E and vitamin C.

- Reduces inflammation of liver and spleen. It will relieve symptoms associated with liver disease, such as itching, nausea, poor appetite, bloating, and insomnia. It also lowers cholesterol levels.

- Protects the liver against severely toxic chemicals which harm the levels of glutathione.

- Helps to repair damaged liver cells and restore liver function. It prevents toxins from entering liver cells and encourages the growth of new liver cells. It is recommended to take silymarin if you happen to be taking harsh herbs or drugs.

Take milk thistle as a tincture of the powdered seed, as powder, or in food. It usually takes numerous capsules to make an effective dose. If you are an herb gatherer, you may find your own milk thistle growing on disturbed ground. Harvest the seeds when the flowers have turned to little white parachutes.

## Melatonin and Honokiol for Sleep

These two supplements may be the most important of all, a lifesaver for people who have trouble sleeping. Taken before bed, they make it easier to sleep.

Melatonin, a hormone produced in the pineal gland, regulates circadian rhythms and our response to light and dark, telling us when to sleep and when to wake. Light inhibits production of melatonin, whereas darkness promotes it. It is also an antioxidant and is thought to have a part in production of the T lymphocytes of the immune system. Research suggests that melatonin has anti-aging properties. Besides its beneficial effects for immune disorders, it is valuable for depression and insomnia. If you wake up at least 4 hours before you want to get up, it is okay to take another dose.

**Honokiol from magnolia bark** (*Magnolia grandiflora*) can noticeably decrease anxiety and depression. Since it can cause substantial drowsiness, it is a good adjunct to melatonin as a sleep aid. When taken during the day it is very calming.

# Medicinal Spices

*Why would a man die whilst sage grows in his garden?*

Medieval proverb

These five herbs, turmeric, garlic, ginger, capsicum, and green tea appear in many ethnic medical systems and cuisines. They offer serious dynamic support in any healing program. All may be consumed as foods and spices but are also available in capsules. They are herbs to take on a daily basis.

**Handy tool:** Use a "Cap-M-Quik" capsule roller to make "OO" or other size capsules of powdered turmeric, ginger, capsicum, and other medicinal herbs at home. Powders are available in bulk from natural food stores or other suppliers.

## Turmeric (*Curcumin*)

Turmeric has a 5,000 year history as a healer in the Ayurvedic system of medicine. It is a tropical rhizome related to ginger and cardamom and is the main ingredient in curry powder. It is a major medicinal herb and is totally nontoxic.

- Turmeric stimulates the immune system and aids in adrenal hormone function.

- Besides repairing the liver, it can increase glutathione levels.

- It protects against the formation of ulcers, although large doses may promote ulcers.

- Turmeric inhibits gas formation and intestinal spasm.

- It prevents the formation of atherosclerosis.

- It is comparable to vitamin C as an antioxidant. As a scavenger of free radicals it is more efficient than lipoic acid, vitamin E, or beta-carotene.

- It has the ability to block chemicals such as pesticides from invading cells.

- It also serves as an anti-depressant and nerve protector.

- The active ingredient, curcumin, is similar to cortisone, but much safer in its effect on acute inflammation and rheumatoid arthritis. Though it is half as effective, it does not have the terrible side effects that cortisone has.

• Turmeric is also antiasthmatic.

If you take prescription drugs, it is best to take the curcumin two hours away from them.

Use turmeric liberally as a spice with meals. Assimilation of turmeric can increase twenty fold if taken with a little black pepper.[64]

**Caution**: Curcumin should not be taken on an empty stomach as it can cause discomfort.

## Garlic: Secret of the Four Thieves

**Garlic** is one of nature's most valuable healers. During the plague of 1721, four famous thieves robbed corpses, escaping the plague by fortifying themselves with "Four Thieves' Vinegar"— garlic macerated in wine.

**Onions** have many of the same qualities that garlic has. The Egyptians regarded the onion, because of its many layers, as a symbol of the universe. It is also a metaphor for healing. As one layer heals, a deeper layer will present itself.

In countries where garlic consumption is high, cancer rates are low. In sufficient quantities it can protect against cancer, particularly in the gastro-intestinal tract, and destroy potent bacteria, viruses, fungus, and parasites. It kills only harmful bacteria while at the same time enhancing friendly flora. It is called "Russian penicillin" because it was used as an antiseptic and antibiotic in both world wars. Albert Schweitzer used it in Africa against amoebic dysentery.

Mark Konlee reports that seven AIDS patients took 5 cloves of garlic daily as aged extract. After six weeks, six of them had normal NK cell activity, and all had normal NK cell activity after 12 weeks. In those who ate two bulbs a day NK cell activity increased by 140%. Those who consumed 1800 mg of odorless aged garlic a day saw increases of 156%.[65]

- Garlic compares in effectiveness to pharmaceuticals in lowering cholesterol and fighting fungus infections. It reduces atherosclerosis and platelet aggregation and is more effective as an antifungal than gentian violet or nystatin.

- It reduces clotting (fibrinolytic), and it can lower blood pressure.

- It aids digestion, relieving flatulence, nausea, vomiting, colic, and indigestion.

- Besides being a powerful anti-microbial, garlic will also oxidize heavy metals and make them soluble in water for easy elimination. Its biologically active natural selenium defends against mercury poisoning.

Garlic is best used raw, immediately, because its allicin content will deteriorate rapidly. You can also use freeze dried garlic supplement or tincture. Eat raw garlic with other foods, rather than alone. It is best to start with small amounts and build up to a therapeutic dose (five or more cloves of raw garlic a day or its equivalent in capsules).

The stronger the smell of garlic, the greater is its healing quality. Chewing on parsley will minimize garlic breath. Juice a clove of garlic when you make your carrot juice. Put garlic or garlic tincture on food three times a day. Use garlic liberally in sauces. When garlic is used with other herbs its potency can increase up to six fold.

## Capsicum

Cultures that use cayenne or capsicum liberally report lower rates of cardiovascular disease due to its action in reducing blood cholesterol, triglyceride levels, and platelet aggregation. It is a remedy for asthma, fever, respiratory infections, and digestive disturbances; It thins mucus; It fights bacteria; It increases fibrinolytic activity, making it useful in treating biofilms and cancer.

If you are rolling it into caps, be aware of the potency and be cautious with it. It is available in different BTUs (levels of heat). If you take too much it can cause temporary distress. Add a little cayenne to juices and smoothies. Build up to whatever quantity you can tolerate. See Sam Biser's book, *A Layman's Guide to Curing with Cayenne and its Herbal Partners*, for some remarkable healing suggestions using cayenne.

## Green Tea (*Camellia sinensis*)

Green tea represents all that is most delicate and mysterious, and at the same time, most strong and energizing in Japanese culture. Daily use of green tea is thought to be responsible for the low cancer rates in Japan.

- As an antioxidant, the polyphenols in green tea are stronger than vitamins C and E. They increase the activity of glutathione.

- Polyphenols prevent plaque buildup on teeth, improving health of the gums.

- Continued consumption of green tea over time can significantly reduce bad lipoproteins and increase good lipoproteins.

- Green tea improves liver function.

- It has beneficial effects on leukemia.

The valuable ingredients in green tea are the polyphenols catechin, epicatechin, epicatechin gallate, and epigallocatechin gallate, most active in leaf bud and first leaves; and proanthocyanidins. When buying green tea, it is important to be sure that it contains these polyphenols: not all green teas are equal.

To make tea steep one or two teaspoons of green tea per cup of hot water, and drink up to three cups a day. If you prefer to take it in capsules of standardized extract, look especially for epigallocatechin gallate (EGCG) content, though all the compounds in green tea work synergistically.

# Ginger

Ginger is a major herb in the Chinese pharmacopoeia.

- It is a most effective tonic for the gastrointestinal system; it is antispasmodic to the smooth muscle of the GI tract and it helps to prevent ulcers.

- Fresh ginger as a proteolytic enzyme is as effective as the enzymes in papaya and pineapple.

- It increases secretion and excretion of bile, thus helping to lower cholesterol.

- As a remedy for motion sickness it is superior to Dramamine, although larger quantities of it are required for the same effect.

- Ginger is anti-inflammatory.

- Like garlic and onions, ginger is a blood thinner and an antioxidant.

- Fresh ginger is a cardiac tonic.

- Ginger helps to maintain body temperature by facilitating sweating.

For dizziness, nausea and vomiting take 2 teaspoons of dry ginger root powder in hot water or chew on ¼ inch slice of fresh ginger. As an anti-inflammatory for rheumatoid arthritis, the dose would be 3 to 7 grams. Do not take more than 6 grams if your stomach is empty.

## Ethnic Spices

Curry spices not only assist digestion, they have also been shown to inhibit platelet aggregation, fight pathogens, prevent cholesterol absorption from food, and to have fibrinolytic properties.[66] They work together for stronger effect. They include:

| | | |
|---|---|---|
| Cumin Seeds | Cayenne | Fennel |
| Anise | Nutmeg | Black pepper |
| Mace | Cinnamon | Cloves |
| Cardamom | Asafoetida | Fenugreek |
| Turmeric | Basil leaves | Paprika |
| Ginger | Licorice | Orange and lemon peel |

Italian seasoning herbs have antioxidant and antibacterial properties. Their essential oils, notably those of rosemary, oregano, mint, and sage are strong antimicrobials. Many of them, particularly sage, are a liver tonic, blood builder, brain food, and stomach tonic. Use these herbs as much as possible in cooking:

| Parsley | Lemon balm (*Melissa officinalis*) | Oregano |
| Sage (*Salvia officinalis*) | Pepper-mint and spearmint | Marjoram |
| Basil | Rosemary | Thyme |

## Personal Comment

They say charity begins at home. So does healing. To the detriment of total healing, I suspect that the kitchen has been replaced by the laboratory and that supplements are often used as a substitute for good nutrition. Almost every area of the country has wild herbs that are more powerful than any drug. Where I live I have free access to Oregon grape root, stinging nettles, Japanese knotweed, and teasel, for example. It is easy to make tinctures and avoid the escalating costs of supplements if you also eat vital, unprocessed foods.

# NINE

# Spirochetes Hate Heat

*Give me a chance to create a fever and I will cure any disease.*

Parmenides

**Warmth**: Warmth is the medium of growth, of healing, and of energy.

## First Aid for Lyme

Heat therapies are a first line of relief when antibiotics have stopped working and you are feeling as miserable as before (or worse). Heat curbs populations of spirochetes and other organisms associated with Lyme. Hot tubs, steam rooms, and/or saunas will stimulate your body in so many ways that you will start to feel good again. Just a few days of intensive use of hot tubs can have a dramatic effect on overall well-being. For these reasons some people use heat on a daily basis.

## Desperate Heat Treatments and Lyme

The relationship between body temperature and health has been known since ancient times. Heat as a healing practice is probably as ancient as the human race. The Native American sweat lodge is one of the most powerful natural heat therapies known. Science has entered the heat therapy field with whole body hyperthermia, a controversial practice available in Germany, that sedates the patient for a few days and subjects his body to intense heat, causing a massive healing response. It is reported to cure Lyme entirely (if it doesn't kill the patient first). If I had $25,000 in spare change I might consider it.

Treatment with high temperatures initiated by deliberate infection with malaria was once popular in the late 19th century and early 20th century as a cure for late manifestations of systemic syphilis, another well-known spirochete disease. This was a tricky proposition, for while it offered a 30% chance of complete remission, it also offered a 30% chance of death.[67] Lyme desperados have also tried this treatment, but going to Mexico to be injected with blood from a person with malaria is even more hazardous today because of the chance of picking up an HIV infection from that blood.

The good news is that one does not need to go to Germany and spend a fortune or go to Mexico to be infected with malaria: heat therapies may be practiced at home without any possibility of dire consequences. They may not be as dramatic as these desperate therapies, but they are "slo' but sho'."

## Low Thyroid Function and Low Body Temperature in Illness

According to Dr. Broda Barnes,[68] a basal body temperature that stays below 97.8° suggests low thyroid function. This can show itself in symptoms such as coldness, constipation, easy weight gain, heavy periods, elevated blood lipids, mental confusion and depression, hypoglycemia, and increased risk of cancer or diabetes. The key to the body's production of energy is thyroxin, produced by the thyroid gland with the help of iodine (from seaweeds or supplements). Restoring the thyroid to working order is a necessary step in healing.

I have heard claims that high doses of iodine can cure Lyme. Dr. Klinghardt regards iodine as the most critical element for Lyme. High doses of iodine need to be used with care if Hashimoto's thyroiditis is present. Iodine can increase the autoimmune attack on the thyroid gland by intensifying activity of the enzyme thyroid peroxidase, leading to increased inflammation within the thyroid gland. If iodine is to be used in Lyme disease, first ask for a blood test for thyroid peroxidase and anti-thyroglobulin antibodies to rule out Hashimoto's. A properly functioning thyroid is a very good thing.

## Factors That Can Cause Low Body Temperature

Low body temperature accompanies poor resistance to chronic illness. Some of the causative factors of low body temperature are:

- Low amino acid levels caused by eating primarily processed foods. This may be remedied by eating whole foods and taking amino acid supplements.

- Toxic metals such as lead. Garlic, chlorophyll from green plants, especially cilantro, and pectin from citrus rinds (fresh or powdered) will remove heavy metals.

## Effects of Low Body Temperature

- Low production of energy (ATP)

- Low hormone levels from pituitary, thyroid and adrenal glands, low output of enzymes from liver and pancreas, and poor kidney function

- Poor removal of toxins from bloodstream

- Further depression of body temperature leading to progression of disease

- Poor absorption of herbs and other supplements, especially B12, leading to increased mental dysfunction and neuropathy

## Heat Shock Response and *Borrelia Burgdorferi*

"Heat shock response" occurs when sub-lethal high temperature activates "heat shock proteins" or "stress proteins."[69] The heat shock response is valuable because it increases the power of the immune system to recognize foreign bacteria, bind heat shock proteins to antigens, and fight the invader. It helps the body to recognize stressors such as infection, inflammation, exercise, exposure to toxins and heavy metals, ultraviolet light, nutritional starvation, oxygen starvation, or water deprivation,[70] and calms them. Chronic fatigue syndrome and fibromyalgia improve with toxin removal through the heat shock response, especially when missing minerals and other nutrients are replenished.

In vitro cultivation of *B. burgdorferi* reveals that the spirochete replicates most quickly at 37°C (98.6°F, normal body temperature). An increase in temperature to 39°C (102°F) can considerably retard its growth, while a 24 hour exposure at 41°C (106°F) kills all spirochetes in the culture. This reveals that the optimal growth temperature of *B. burgdorferi* is only 4°C below the upper lethal limit." [71]

In practice this suggests that a temperature high enough to kill Lyme bacteria might also kill the Lyme person. But temporary application of temperatures of 102° F, 103° F, or 104° F. will definitely make the organisms want to leave the comforts your body has provided for them. At the very least these temperatures would cut them down to size for a while.

Besides killing spirochetes, temporary fevers assist the immue system in other ways:

• Metabolism and pulse rates increase.

• T-cells and antibodies can increase by up to 2000%.

• White blood cells become more mobile and active in killing bacteria.

• Circulation and oxygen delivery to the cells increases.

• Tumor necrosis factor increases by up to 500 times.

- Sweat removes more chemical and heavy metal toxins than urine does.

- Muscles relax.

- Calcium deposits and scar tissue in blood vessel walls are broken down.

# Heat Therapy for Detoxification[72]

The effectiveness of heat and/or water therapies arises from their action on the blood and lymph channels. Since lymph fluid can make up as much as a third of total body weight, it is a primary route for removal of toxins. The lymph system contains about 45 ounces of lymph fluid compared to the blood system's fifteen ounces of blood. Lymph flows directly under the skin making it easily responsive to applications of heat. Stimulating the lymph will affect all the tissues of the body.

## Considerations in Using Heat Therapies

- Use common sense—start cautiously, as you may experience dizziness, headache, exhaustion, nausea, nervousness, aches and pains, insomnia, palpitations, faintness or chilliness.  You need to know what you can handle and what is best for your condition. Since high heat could create a sizable Herxheimer response, a sensible approach would be to start slowly and build up as tolerance to heat increases.

- Intensive heat therapies should be done under competent advisement.

- Heating and sweating may be contraindicated in anemia, debilitation, asthma, heart problems, severe colds, diabetes, dizziness, pregnancy, and acute bladder infection.

- Heat dilates the blood vessels, but too much heat leads to stagnation. Sessions should not be prolonged beyond com-mon-sense limits.

- While using heat therapies, drink fresh juices, lemon juice, green tea and plenty of water to flush out toxins. The potas-sium in fresh juices will help you sweat. Yarrow tea will be of particular help with sweating.

## Dry Heat

Infrared saunas are the best first aid for flare-ups of Lyme, chron-ic fatigue, and fibromyalgia. Without sufficient far-infrared light from the sun we suffer depression and other illnesses. In the far-infrared (FIR) sauna, we take in only infrared wave lengths without ultraviolet rays or other harmful radiation. Some of the metabo-lic effects of sunlight and far-infrared saunas are similar to those achieved with exercise.

FIR heat bestows all the benefits of an artificial fever. When subjected to heat, the water molecules of the body vibrate and break down, releasing toxic matter. Conventional saunas release 95-97% water, while infrared saunas release 80-85% water, releasing at the same time cholesterol, fat-soluble toxins, heavy metals, and envi-ronmental toxins such as pesticides and herbicides. Infrared sau-nas may be used as an alternative therapy for mercury detoxifica-tion. They are up to seven times more effective at detoxification of mercury and heavy metals than conventional saunas. Infrared radiant heat can penetrate the body to a depth of 1.5 inches. Some manufacturers claim their units can penetrate even deeper.

The commercial wood infrared sauna contains heating ele-ments coated with space-age far-infrared radiant materials which are activated by heat. If you purchase one of these wooden saunas, be sure they are "low EMF," low electro-magnetic frequency. This applies also if you purchase tent-type FIR saunas.

Directions for making a sauna tent with infrared bulbs rather than space-age materials may be obtained from L. D. Wilson's *Sauna Therapy for Detoxification and Healing*. I made one of these for about $100 following his directions. I can vouch for its ability to cause sweating. It is important to get the type of infrared bulbs recommended in the book. I include here some comments I received regarding infrared bulbs from my friend Rob Abramowitz, an engineer.

## Selecting an Infrared Sauna, by Rob Abramowitz

Many disease agents (viruses and bacteria) cannot stand heat. That is why we get fevers when we get sick: it is our body's way of trying to fight the disease. Just being in a hot environment, though, does not raise our internal body temperature. Our perspiration keeps our body cool inside. Infrared saunas can take advantage of the temperature sensitivity of diseases through the beneficial effects of:

- Sweating out toxins

- Directly killing off bacteria/viruses/spirochetes

Various kinds of dry heat saunas can be used to aid in sweating out toxins, but only infrared saunas can directly kill off viruses/bacteria/spirochetes. This is because the infrared light can penetrate the skin and directly affect the disease causing agent. The remainder of this paper is about infrared saunas.

Unfortunately, there is much misunderstanding of infrared technology. In order to understand better how to choose an infrared sauna, it may help to understand how light interacts with the skin.

Our skin is opaque to the light we can see with our eyes. If it were not, we would be like some translucent fishes where we could see each other's' internal organs. Our skin blocks visible light and prevents us from seeing what's inside us. Our skin blocks most light within 1/20 inch. The exception is infrared light. Some infrared light can penetrate up to 1/2 inch. This allows infrared light to reach our blood circulatory system in which disease agents travel.

But not all infrared light is able to penetrate the skin. Near infrared light is little better than visible light at penetrating the skin. What is called middle infrared light is the most effective at penetrating the skin and reaching the disease agents. In technical terms the light we can see has a wavelength of about 390 nm (blue) -750 nm (red) (note, nm stands for nanometer, and billionths of a meter which is about .00000004 inches). Near infrared light extends from 750 nm to about 1000 nm. This near infrared light does not penetrate the skin much more than visible light. It is only when we get to the middle infrared (technically high-near infrared) that light penetrates the skin. The most effective infrared light for penetrating the skin is between 1500 nm to 3000 nm. This light is far beyond anything that the eye can perceive.

This last fact can be very helpful in selecting appropriate saunas: if the heating element visibly glows, then the light given off by the element will probably not penetrate the skin well. That is, if a sauna or a heating lamp has an element that glows visibly, then it is not going to be useful for directly killing off disease agents. Some manufacturers try to get around this issue by either hiding the elements from direct view or by using deep red bulbs or filters. Hiding the heating element greatly reduces its efficiency. Putting a red filter over the element just eliminates the glare of the visible light; it does not increase the infrared light. So, if you can't see the heating elements or if there is a red filter over the elements, don't buy it.

Even in this golden area of 1500 nm to 3000 nm, only about 1% of light makes it through the skin and into the circulatory system. In order to overcome this, you will need lots and lots of infrared light. If this is a whole body sauna, I suggest at least 1200 W or more (10 amps at 120 V). Some manufacturers make infrared systems for the hand or arm only. These probably should have at least 250 W of power.

Some manufacturers are using LEDs. In general they do not use

LEDs that are of the right wavelength. If you find one that does specify somewhere in the golden range of 1500 nm to 3000 nm, make sure that it emits at least 250 W.

Many patients are using bathroom type infrared lamps to create an infrared sauna. These lamps radiate mostly in the visible light range and very little in the middle infrared range. They are ineffective as infrared saunas. As a general rule of thumb:

- If you can't see the heating elements don't buy it.

- If the bulb or elements have a red filter, don't buy it.

- If the heating elements visibly glow, don't buy it.

- A good element for an infrared sauna should warm up very slowly and take many minutes to feel very warm.

I hope this was of some help. My own personal experience has found infrared saunas to be extremely helpful in my own fight against Lyme disease.

## Detoxification Baths[73]

Soaking in a bathtub of 105° to 107° F is an easy way to increase body temperature. The pulse should be under 72 when you start, and should not be allowed to get above 90. Count the pulse with fingers beside the larynx at the side of the neck for one minute.

Detoxification baths may be taken three or more times a week. Before getting in a tub full of hot water, have a basin of ice water close by, a wet towel to cool your forehead as needed, and water to drink. Cover the upper drain of the tub with duct tape so you can have more water in the tub. You can monitor your body temperature by keeping a thermometer in your mouth while you are in the tub. You can stay in the bath for an hour, keeping the temperature hot, around 104°. Do not let your body temperature go above 104°. Use a cold compress to prevent headache. Shower when you are done. Wrap yourself in a clean sheet and lie down to cool off slowly.

Be careful, especially if you feel dizzy.

## Epsom Salt (Magnesium Sulfate) Baths and Foot Baths

Caution: Epsom salt baths are contraindicated for persons who have high blood pressure or heart conditions. Those who are frail or elderly or those who have difficulty moving their joints without excessive pain can start with ¼ cup of Epsom salts and gradually increase the amount. The Epsom Salt Industry Council lists the following benefits[74] of Epsom salts:

- Reduces irregular heartbeats, prevents hardening of the arteries, reduces blood clots and lowers blood pressure.

- Improves the use of insulin, reducing the incidence or severity of diabetes.

- Removes toxins and heavy metals from the cells, easing muscle pain.

- Regulates electrolytes for better nerve function, and maintains proper calcium levels in the blood.

- Relieves stress by binding adequate amounts of serotonin for mood elevation.

- Reduces inflammation to relieve pain and muscle cramps.

- Improves oxygen use in the body.

- Improves absorption of nutrients.

- Prevents or eases migraine headaches.

### Directions

1. Start with ¼ cup of Epsom salts. In subsequent baths, gradually build up to 4 cups per bath. Soak for 15 minutes. Do

not use soap in an Epsom salts bath.

2. While in the bath keep a cool wet hand towel wrapped around your neck and drink plenty of cool filtered water.

3. When you have finished, take a cool shower or sponge bath.

4. Lie down and rest for at least 15 to 30 minutes after the bath.

## Floatation Tanks

Floatation tank sessions offer a very effective way to absorb quantities of magnesium through the skin. The concentration of magnesium in the water is so strong that the body floats on the surface of the solution with the face out of the water. Floating in these tanks is also a very meditative experience, since all sensory input from the outside is eliminated. The float is so peaceful that many people doze off. Regular sessions can provide substantial relief from chronic stress-related ailments such as anxiety, depression and fibromyalgia. In recent studies more than three quarters of the subjects experienced noticeable improvements.[75] Positive effects remained even four months after the treatment ended. Sessions are available for a fee from some wellness centers.

## Wet Sauna

A home tent sauna or steam cabinet, where heat is supplied by a steam cooker, can have a stimulating effect on the lymph system. These tent saunas may be used also for ozone sauna treatments.

## Finnish Dry or Steam Sauna

The dry sauna increases sweating. Start with 5-minute sessions and build up to 30 minutes, but no longer. Drink plenty of fluid, and shower when done.

## Using Hot Packs

If a deep bathtub is not available, placing hot packs such as hydro-collator packs on the body and wrapping yourself in blankets can achieve a similar heating effect. Hydrocollator packs are heated clay packs used by chiropractors to relax tense muscles. It is not necessary to buy the automatic hydrocollator heating unit, but it is important to have hot enough water (160º) to soak the packs. Place the hot packs in special pads to prevent burns. Or just cover the packs with towels and avoid buying the covers. Hot packs applied over lymphatic areas can provide relief from lymph congestion.[76] Lymph congestion may also be relieved by castor oil packs placed over affected areas.

# TEN

# Cellular Respiration

*In the treatment of the sick person, the physician must be free to use*
*a new diagnostic or therapeutic measure, if in his or her judgment it*
*offers hope of saving life, re-establishng health or alleviating suffering.*

Adopted by the 18th World Medical Assembly, Helsinki, Finland, June 1964

**Essential Elements of Life**: Oxygen is the second most abundant element on Earth. It is renewed and replenished by the photosynthesis of plants and algae. Oxygen is the crucial element required for cellular respiration in our bodies.

## Fibromyalgia and Chronic Fatigue: Disorders of Oxygen Metabolism?

ATP, the primary energy source in the body, is generated by oxygen. Dr. Majid Ali states that it is the accumulation of toxins in neurons and nerve fibers combined with lack of functional oxygen that is the cause of neuropathy. He says this is the result of "sticky sugars, rancid fats, mangled proteins, and others."[77] This means that sufficient oxygen in the body, acting in a detergent function, can prevent and control neuropathy. Ali finds it deplorable that neurologists do not acknowledge toxicities or oxygen therapies.

Dr. Ali claims that both chronic Lyme disease and fibromyalgia are disorders of oxygen metabolism in the body. That which starts out as oxygen deficiency becomes compounded by the resulting buildup of acids and thickening of bodily fluids, leading to further oxygen deficits and debility. According to Dr. Ali, the cumulative effect of oxygen deficiency is felt in trigger points where the muscles are tight and painful. He found that chronic Lyme persons had high urinary organic acids—a result of oxygen dysfunction. Dysfunctional oxygen metabolism stems from a failure of the enzymes involved in oxygen metabolism. He calls this his ODD (oxidative-dysoxygenative dysfunction) theory of the fibromyalgia/fatigue complex. Ali says that the longer patients are on antibiotics the sicker they grow. Patients can reverse this situation by working to correct their bowel, liver, thyroid, and adrenal problems. Exceptions to this are persons with exceptionally difficult life situations or deep, unresolved anger and depression.[78]

His method of dealing with neuropathy consists of:

Hydrogen peroxide foot soaks

Castor oil rub

Antifungal herbs and drugs in rotation to control gut fermentation

Six-week trial of gluten-free, sugar-free, dairy-free diet

B vitamin supplementation along with B12 injections

Magnesium, potassium, calcium and sometimes lipoic acid supplementation

Chelation of toxic metals

# Oxygen Deprivation is Responsible for the Four Primary Symptoms of Fibromyalgia

- Persistent muscle pain and weakness

- Disabling fatigue

- Brain fog (problems of mood, memory, and mentation)

- Air hunger

## Other Symptoms of Oxygen Deprivation

- Immune system symptoms such as sore throats, swollen glands, pain in the tissues

- Abdominal bloating, cramps, diarrhea, constipation, poor digestion, and malabsorption of nutrients

- Sensitivity to cold

- Poor circulation

- Sleep difficulties and restless leg syndrome

- Dizziness, heart palpitations, and irregular heartbeats

- Dryness of skin, eyes, mouth, and vaginal tissues

- Vaginitis, bladder spasms, and bladder infections in women and prostatitis in men

- Joint and muscle stiffness and pain

- Lack of sex drive in both sexes and menstrual irregularities in women

## How Lack of Oxygen Depletes Energy

Red blood cells carry oxygen to cells to produce energy and carbon dioxide to the lungs to be exhaled. An oxygen environment in the blood inhibits growth of bacteria and viruses, whereas excess carbon dioxide in the blood increases acidity and reduces the level of available oxygen (hypoxia). Oils rich in omega-3 fatty acids increase the power of the blood to carry oxygen and combat viruses, cancers, and microbes. Another way to keep the level of carbon dioxide down is to increase the alkalinity of the blood through raw fruits, vegetables, and juices.

Depletion of oxygen leads to depletion of energy. When there is sufficient oxygen in the blood, glucose breaks down into carbon dioxide and water, resulting in high energy gain. Insufficient oxygen turns it into lactic acid and water, producing only small energy gains. As ATP levels increase, energy and heat increase. The formula for normal cell respiration shows the body's need for sufficient oxygen:

$C_6H_{12}O_6$ + 6 $O_2$ → 6 $CO_2$ + 6 $H_2O$ + ATP (energy)

Glucose + oxygen → carbon dioxide + water + 2870 kjoules

Insufficient oxygen will prevent this equation from happening properly. Just one less molecule of oxygen changes the equation:

$C_6H_{12}O_6$ + 5 $O_2$ → 4 $CO_2$ + 6 $H_2O$ + 2 CO + ATP

Glucose + oxygen→ carbon dioxide + water + carbon monoxide +2500 kjoules

The cell is slowly poisoning itself. Further along, the equation becomes cancer. Notice that the energy level is 20 times less than in the normal cell.

$C_6H_{12}O6$ → $2C_3H_5O_3$ + 2 H + ATP

Fermentation of glucose→ lactic acid + hydrogen ions + 150 kjoules

I quote directly from Dr. Saul Pressman[79]

1. Free radical formation is not related to oxygen in the body. Rather it is related to a buildup of toxins that prevent the normal protective enzymes from doing their work. If there are no toxins, there is no damage, because of the elegant design of the cell. It is the failure to maintain a clean environment that causes the problem, not the oxygen. You might as well say that eating causes free radicals. Just as informative and just as useless.

2. If singlet oxygen $O_1$ finds another singlet oxygen $O_1$, it will form $O_2$, which is less reactive than $O_1$.

3. DNA is protected by the enzymes in the cell. Oxygen is not mutagenic.

4. Oxidative damage of cells does NOT cause cancer. Rather, a LACK of oxygen causes cancer because of the fall back

mechanism in every cell allowing it to ferment sugar when it cannot get sufficient oxygen to burn the sugar. Once the cell has been chronically starved for oxygen and in the fermentative mode, it is EXTREMELY difficult to convert it back to normal oxidative mode. Instead, it is headed on the road to becoming a cancer cell. If it is stimulated by enzyme growth factors, secreted by T-cells in response to the acidity surrounding a fermenting cell (waste is lactic acid), it will begin to replicate wildly, starting off a vicious circle of growth → acidity → enzyme growth factors → growth. The only thing that will interrupt this cycle is to oxidize the lactic acid (ozone) and/or destroy the cell (ozone).

5. Aging is related to toxic buildup, not to oxidative damage. Several scientists have been able to keep chicken cells in vitro living for over 60 years, through the simple means of providing adequate oxygen, nutrients and waste disposal. As soon as the wastes were allowed to build up, the cells died. Oxidative damage had nothing to do with it. Rather, a LACK of oxidation allowed the buildup of garbage, which inhibited cell operation, and caused aging and death. Normal cells have their own built-in protection against reactive oxygen species (ROS): superoxide dismutase (SOD), glutathione peroxidase, catalase (specific for hydrogen peroxide) and reductase. They are unable to work when the system is overloaded with toxins. Eliminating the toxins and raising pH will return this condition to normal.

# Ozone

## The Rationale for Oxygen Therapies

No disease stands alone: factors that contribute to one disease also contribute to another. In 1931 Otto Warburg won the Nobel Prize for discovering that "cancer has only one prime cause. It is the replacement of normal oxygen respiration of the body's cells by an

anaerobic (i.e. oxygen-deficient) cell respiration."[80] And in this connection he said cancer is also dependent upon fermenting sugars in
the blood which are incompletely broken down by a system lacking
oxygen. Lyme spirochetes, other microbes, and fungi also feed on
sugar.

High oxygen concentration in the blood is needed for enzyme
production in the liver and for detoxification in general. The quantity of toxins excreted by Lyme spirochetes can lead to marked depletion of oxygen levels in the body. The resulting acidity is treated
by the white blood cells as a signal that an injury needs to be re-
paired by cell proliferation.

In the case of cancer, increasing oxygenation is the first step
in reversing it because cancer cannot live in the presence of an adequate supply of oxygen.[81] A proper supply of oxygen in the blood
breaks down the fermenting sugars upon which cancer depends
(the Krebs cycle). Since Lyme disease also feasts on, prospers, and
makes itself at home when fed a diet rich in too much sugar, ozone
would be a first-choice therapy to consider for maintaining oxygen
levels in the body.

## Ozone: An Easy Way to Get More Oxygen into the Body

The ozone generator was invented by Nikola Tesla over 100
years ago. Ozone has been used in medicine ever since, although
the medical establishment in this country has been reluctant to
recognize it.

I have found ozone treatments which I do at home to be a most
effective and stabilizing self-healing therapy. Ozone is easy to do
and does not require heroic efforts. I have been doing this for almost fifteen years with the same ozone generator. I have learned to
be consistent with it (though it took me ten years to comprehend
that consistency is the key to effectiveness). Ozone forestalls bad
flare-ups under normal circumstances. I have found persons on the

web who claim to have cured their Lyme by doing ozone saunas twice a day along with other home delivery methods. Whether you have this sort of discipline or not, ozone should be a part of every day in some form or other.

## Mistaken Beliefs about Ozone

1. Ozone is not smog. Ozone is nature's method of cleaning the atmosphere. Its presence in smog is nature's attempt to clean up man's mess. Ozone cannot be produced inside the internal combustion engine: it is produced when sunlight hits pollutants in the air. If there were more ozone there would be less of a problem, because all of the pollutants would be broken down into their constituents. Carbon monoxide is one of the worst constituents of smog. Ozone transforms it into harmless carbon dioxide.

2. Ozone is a not radical new-age experiment. Ozone therapy has been practiced since 1870. It is presently used in 24 countries by thousands of doctors. Millions of people have been safely and effectively treated with ozone therapy through various delivery techniques.

3. Ozone is not something you breathe. Breathing ozone is not a medical therapy, as the lungs cannot tolerate pure ozone.

4. Ozone/oxygen is not a free radical. As oxygen is fed through an ozone machine it absorbs electrons, forming $O_3$ or $O_4$. $O_3$ breaks down into $O_2$ and $O_1$ in the presence of water, releasing these electrons into the water. The difference between $O_3$ and hydrogen peroxide, $H_2O_2$, in terms of reactivity is these free electrons. Ozone actually destroys free radicals that are trying to take electrons from healthy cells.

## Medical Ozone Machines

The primary producer of ozone for clinical and home use is the high-frequency cold plasma ozone generator which converts oxygen into ozone. Oxygen is fed into this machine from an oxygen tank equipped with a pediatric oxygen regulator calibrated from 0 to 4 liters per minute with settings beginning at 1/32 LPM. Another dial regulates output of ozone from the ozone generator. The ozone comes out through silicone tubing for delivery to the desired application.

Once you have an ozone generator the only expense involved is the replenishment of your oxygen tank once in a while. I use oxygen from a welding shop, and this runs about $15-$20 for a 40-lb. tank which can last for many months, depending on use. Oxygen from a welding supply house is the same as oxygen from a medical supplier but is much less expensive than the medical oxygen.

Ozone generators can run from $1,000 to $3,500 with all the trimmings. A cheap machine is available from China which seems to be a decent enough machine except that it emits a very distracting high-pitched whine.

Machines that obtain oxygen from ambient air (room purifying machines) also emit nitrogen, which is not desirable for most medical ozone applications. These room-air machines are, however, adequate for use with the ozone sauna or for making ozonated water.

## Effects of Ozone Therapies [82]

- The primary effect of ozone therapies is to stimulate production of enzymes which scavenge excess free radicals.

- Ozone oxidizes the toxins which keep the normal free-radical-scavenger enzymes from cleaning up free radicals.

- Ozone stimulates the immune system by enhancing production of gamma interferon, interleukin 2, NK killer cells, and T-cells.

- Ozone destroys bacteria and viruses.

- Ozone increases the production of tumor necrosis factor, acting as an anti-cancer agent.

- Ozone therapy keeps blood cells from sticking together. When blood cells stick together they cannot get through the small capillaries. This is what happens in diabetes. Platelets can act as a glue that allows cancer cells to stick to the walls of blood vessels (platelet aggregation).

- Ozone increases tissue oxygenation.

- Ozone accelerates the citric acid cycle, the main cycle for liberating energy from sugars, stimulating basic metabolism and increasing production of ATP.

## Considerations in the Use of Ozone

Ozone treatments should be done a couple hours before or after eating. Dr. Pressman recommends doing ozone treatments no more than 5 times a week, taking two days off before starting another round of treatment. Oxygen therapy is not advisable if you are taking iron supplements; they react badly together.

## Warnings:

- Too much of oxidating therapies can shut down the immune system. Low quantities of ozone stimulate the immune system, while higher doses will depress it by harming red blood cell membranes. When higher doses are used like antibiotics, this suppressive action will happen.

- Do not breathe pure ozone. It will harm your lungs. If this should occur, the antidote is a large dose of vitamin C. The amount of escaped ozone which you might breathe in the course of treating yourself is generally not harmful where there is good ventilation.

- If you are relying on your own ozone treatments for Lyme, it is imperative to do them regularly forever. It is easy to "forget" to do it when you are feeling good. This forgetfulness can last for months and result in flare-ups. It has to be a regular part of your life.

# Home Methods of Delivery

## Cupping or Funneling

Ozone may be directed to painful or inflamed areas of the body such as over the liver or directly over skin disorders, lymphomas or tumors by means of funneling onto the affected area. You can purchase special ozone suction cups or simply make one at home with a common household funnel attached to ozone-proof tubing. Wet the skin, hold the funnel against the skin, and run low concentration ozone to that area.

## Ozone Sauna (Transdermal Ozone Therapy)

Ozone saunas are powerful, relaxing, and enjoyable to do. They combine the detoxifying effects of the steam sauna with the detoxifying and oxygenating effects of ozone. These saunas are particularly beneficial for the lymph system. The combination of heat, moisture, and ozone makes the sauna a good place for funneling ozone over problem areas.

The ozone sauna can be either a solid plastic stand-alone unit or a fiberglass tent-like apparatus that works with a steam cooker and an ozone generator. The head remains outside the sauna.

When using the ozone sauna, it is recommended that you wrap a towel around your neck to keep you from breathing ozone. You may stay in the sauna for about thirty minutes or until you start to feel the heat shock. Always get out of the sauna if you become dizzy or uncomfortable. Do not do an ozone sauna at night because it is so stimulating that it hinders sleep. All the precautions mentioned for heat therapies also apply here.

Some people report skin itching when doing a series of saunas. This is a result of the detoxifying action of the saunas. Systemic pancreatic enzymes will help with this, as will cutting back on the saunas until the itching improves.

## Insufflations

**Vaginal**: Women have an advantage in being able to do vaginal insufflations. According to Dr. Pressman, these are preferable to rectal insufflations for most purposes. Compliance is better because no colon cleansing is required beforehand. Vaginal insufflations allow the ozone to get into the lymph as well as the blood, making it more beneficial for the whole system. It affects directly such problems as candida, endometriosis, and late period. This should not be done during pregnancy. Use the lowest setting on both pediatric regulator and ozone machine, for up to half an hour at a time.

**Rectal**: Men will need to do rectal insufflations, but for shorter periods. Rectal ozone insufflations will directly affect intestinal problems, and will get ozone into the bloodstream. It has the disadvantage over time of harming some of the good flora, so it is generally used only for serious conditions such as AIDS, ulcerative colitis, or colon cancer: in this case the benefits far outweigh the disadvantage. Though it is generally recommended to do an enema beforehand, one ozone doctor told me that a recent bowel movement will serve just as well.

**Ear**: Persons with Lyme who do ear insufflations usually experience a marked improvement over brain fog and an increase in mental acuity. In order to avoid experiencing dizziness and nausea from doing this too vigorously, start with a few seconds in each ear. Ear insufflations are easy to do: lowest (1/32) concentrations of ozone are gently (very gently) blown into the ear using a small tube or simply placing the connector at the end of the ozone tube into the ear. This will also help clear the sinus areas. Persons who are able to do a regular series of ear insufflations of sufficient duration (after working up very slowly to 15 minutes) have claimed to eradicate their Lyme entirely. Since many people have reported this, it is worth a try.

## Ozonated Water

Ozonated water is particularly useful for stomach, kidney and bladder. It helps digestion and liver, slows collagen breakdown, and reduces the stress and pain of chronic illness. It is a useful adjunct in treating many diseases where blood and lymph could benefit from increased oxygen. Drinking it regularly will improve blood counts and normalize blood pressure and pulse rates. Drink ozonated water on an empty stomach because it can cause nausea if combined with food.

Ozonated water is made by bubbling ozone from your ozone machine through cold, distilled water (ozone dissipates in warmer water) for 5 minutes or more. Drinking several doses of ozonated water during the day is quite safe. The freshly made water should be used immediately as the ozone does not remain in solution for long.

## Skin Bagging

Skin bagging will concentrate ozone on specific limbs, parts of limbs, or even the entire body. You can purchase specially made bags, or you can make do with a plastic bag fastened securely around the area to prevent leaks. First wet the skin, then insert the ozone tube through a small hole in the bag. If you have an ozone destructor to catch any escaping ozone, you will need to make another hole for it. These ozone destructors come with some of the more expensive machines. However, adequate ventilation will take care of any problems with ozone leaking from the bag. I have seen Kaposi sarcomas shrink and become lighter in color after only a half hour of ozone bagging.

# Ozonated Olive Oil

Ozonated olive oil is made by bubbling ozone through extra virgin olive oil for a few weeks until it solidifies. In this state it will keep for long periods of time in the refrigerator. It is better to buy a jar from someone who makes OOO, as it takes a long time and a lot of oxygen to make. It has a powerful effect when applied to the skin, and will help any skin condition. It has also been used for gum conditions.

# One Possible Protocol for Home Ozone Treatments

Ozone can become an early morning ritual. Begin each day with a pint of ozonated water upon arising. If you are taking systemic enzymes, take them with water fifteen minutes after drinking the ozonated water.

When doing several ozone protocols, it is good to make sure you don't forget anything important. Always double check that you have the machine and the oxygen regulator set for your particular use in order to avoid over-or under dosages. Open the oxygen tank valve and turn on the ozone machine (I can't tell you how many times I have forgotten this very important first step). If you are using the ozone sauna, make sure the tubing from the machine is properly attached for ozone to enter the tent.

1. Make ozonated water when you first wake up. Drink it immediately.

2. Start the steamer to heat up the sauna.

3. Do insufflations while waiting for the sauna to get hot. The regulator setting for insufflations is 1/32 LPM and the setting on the ozone generator is the very lowest, setting 1.

4. Follow this with ear insufflations for addressing brain issues. Start slowly with one minute per day in each ear and work

up to 15 minutes in each ear. Dr. Pressman suggests doing this twice a day, but that may be too much for many people.

5. For saunas, turn up ozone concentration, make sure the ozone machine is connected to the sauna, and then get into the sauna. Note that ozone saunas may be done any time during the day except immediately after meals. The time spent in the sauna is a quiet time suitable for meditation or breath work.

6. Get out of the sauna when you feel heat shock starting to happen (it is unmistakable).

7. Close the knob on the oxygen tank and turn off the ozone machine. Disconnect the ozone tubing into the sauna so tubing is available for other uses. Set the pediatric regulator for whatever your next application will require.

8. Shower.

9. Make lemon drink or smoothie or juice.

10. Wait at least half an hour before taking vitamin C or other supplements. Ozone and vitamin C cancel each other out. Likewise, wait at least 6 hours after taking Vitamin C to do ozone.

# Clinical Ozone Treatments

These procedures are probably beneficial for persons who have not yet purchased their ozone machine. The home delivery of rectal insufflations has been reported to be almost as effective as major autohemotherapy.

**Major Autohemotherapy** (MAHT) is widely used in many countries to combat diseases such as hepatitis C, AIDS and some cancers. MAHT involves bubbling ozone through 200 ml of blood which has been withdrawn from the patient. It is then IV dripped back into the blood stream. Some consider this the most valuable oxygen therapy, but home ozone treatments are very effective and enormously cheaper. MAHT is legal in some states here, but doctors who offer it tend to keep a low profile.

**Minor Autohemotherapy** is similar to MAHT, but a much smaller amount of blood is withdrawn for ozonation. The ozonated blood is then injected into the hip.

**Ozonated Saline** is made in a similar fashion by bubbling ozone through saline and then putting it into an intravenous drip. This is a less expensive, less dramatic therapy than MAHT. Some consider it to be just as effective or even more so. It does not require the complicated paraphernalia that MAHT uses.

## Other Types of Home Bio-Oxidative Therapies

**Dilute Hydrogen Peroxide.** Some people have good results drinking a gradually increasing dose of dilute hydrogen peroxide taken in water. Start with one drop and build up gradually to larger doses. As you work up to larger doses it becomes harder to get down because the taste becomes disgusting. This is a serious drawback, as it makes most people give up on it. Use of hydrogen peroxide is also controversial because too much of it can act like a free radical. Hydrogen peroxide is naturally produced in the processes of life in the body and occurs naturally in fruits and vegetables. In small quantities it kills pathogens without causing harm, because catalase enzymes inactivate it. The free radical effect occurs when the catalase is depleted from too large a dose of hydrogen peroxide. A diet high in carotenes (carrot juice) helps to keep the catalase reserves up.

**Hydrogen Peroxide IV drips**, done in a doctor's office. Intravenous diluted hydrogen peroxide gives you a lot of energy and is a serious therapy for serious illness. It is controversial because of the free radical issue.

**Stabilized oxygen** consists of electrolytes of $O_2$, usually in sodium chlorite solution, though some manufacturers now make it with potassium or magnesium solutions. A naturopath from Utah once told me of an HIV positive person who worked up to drinking 50 drops of stabilized oxygen an hour and became symptom free. Always start with just a few drops in water and build up.

# The Effect of Lung Function and Oxygen on Longevity and Illness[83]

The Framingham Study,[84] an ongoing study begun in 1948 and covering thousands of participants, demonstrates that the single most significant factor in staying well and living a long life is how well one breathes—they have proved pulmonary function to be an indicator of "general health and vigor and literally a measure of living capacity.

The best way to bring more oxygen to the cells is to bring more oxygen to the lungs. Lung problems show themselves in shortness of breath, coughing and congestion. Poor lung function contributes to cold hands, weak voice, fatigue, poor sense of smell, excess mucus, sinus problems, airborne allergies, varicose veins, and dry skin. Emotions traditionally associated with poor lung function are grief (due to cells in the body dying from lack of oxygen) attended by hopelessness, sadness, loneliness, and denial. This frequently leads to withdrawal from others. Without sufficient oxygen our life force begins to dwindle away.

The Framingham researchers found they could foretell how long a person would live, even before the person became ill. The study also showed that vital capacity can fall 9 to 27 percent a decade depending on age and sex. Dr. Robert Fried correlates poor breathing habits to many illnesses never before linked to poor breathing.[85]

## EWOT Exercise with Oxygen Therapy

Dr. Manfred von Ardenne, a student of Dr. Otto Warburg, studied the relationship between blood oxygen and illness.[86] He noticed that seriously depleted levels of blood oxygen accompanied illness and shortened life span. He developed what he called an "oxygen multistep therapy" consisting simply of breathing pure oxygen while exercising. It is now generally called EWOT (exercise with oxygen therapy). Commercial sources now advertise exotic exercise machines and personal oxygen generators for this purpose, although most of this is unnecessary. EWOT is a powerful, simple, natural therapy worthy of investigation by anyone who is sick or who would like to avoid becoming sick.

The concept is simple: by breathing higher levels of oxygen while exercising you build greater pressure for driving oxygen into the pulmonary capillaries which, in turn, speeds up the circulation and carries more oxygen to the cells. This process also repairs the mechanism of transfer, ensuring more ongoing diffusion of oxygen to cells that need it.

Von Ardenne believed pulmonary function to be the most important factor in determining whether a person became ill: the more damaged the oxygen transfer mechanism, the greater the possibility of illness. Since this arterial pressure often diminishes with age, anything that would increase it would allow the body to restore younger levels of function. EWOT can do this and, with dedicated effort, can maintain these levels. While EWOT does not claim to be any sort of cure for anything, the higher levels of oxygen can help with:

- Energy levels, strength, and stamina
- Emphysema and other circulatory problems, if practiced regularly
- Cataracts
- Preventing cancer and other illnesses
- Senility, joint problems, liver problems, infections, radiation, strokes, toxins, burns, and stress
- Weight issues
- Decelerating aging

It is commonly accepted that poor mental health is a great contributor to illness and that anything that creates optimism contributes to recovery. When used properly, EWOT can greatly improve the mental predisposition for healing. Improved memory, increased compassion, reduced depression, increased positive thoughts, improved energy, and greater self-awareness will advance any healing process.

Exercise is done on some sort of exercise machine or rebounder while breathing oxygen through an oxygen mask (or cannula or head set) at a flow rate of four to six liters per minute. An intensive EWOT therapy would consist of practicing two hours per day in an 18-day, 36-hour program. However, common sense would dictate working within any individual's capacities. Application should be geared to the condition of the body and should not overwhelm an already impaired system. Taking 30 mg of thiamin (vitamin B1) and 100 mg of magnesium orotate half an hour before beginning exercise will augment the effects of the oxygen.

Persons who are fairly healthy need only exercise for 15 minutes but can increase the rate of oxygen delivery. One can, of course, practice any combination of time and oxygen strength.

## The Set-Up

The simplest way to set up is to purchase an oxygen tank from a welding supply shop, a pediatric regulator to put on the tank, an oxygen mask, and a small rebounder, treadmill or exercise bike. I have found the disposable plastic oxygen masks available in health supply stores to be frustrating to use and too plastic-smelling. A number of websites sell oxygen masks to use with EWOT.

This process uses a lot of oxygen, so a larger tank (maybe 40 lbs.) is preferable to a smaller one. Another option is to use an oxygen concentrator, which supplies oxygen from room air. Though oxygen concentrators do not supply as much oxygen as the simple oxygen tank, they do not need frequent refilling.

# ELEVEN

# Active Breathing

*Breathing is the greatest pleasure in life.*

Giovanni Papini

*This Breathing World: The real energy of our being is lying asleep and inconscient [sic] in the depth of our vital system, and is awakened by the practice of Pranayama.*

Sri Aurobindo

Breathing is the old-fashioned way to get more oxygen into the body. *Pranayama* means "expansion of the breath of life." In the yogic tradition, air is the primary source of prana or life force, a psycho-physio-spiritual force that permeates the universe. Yogic literature tells us that since the breath of life is the food of animate creatures, we should take in as much as possible. The wise ancients regarded the soul as being of the air. In Sanskrit, *atman* means both "breath" and "spirit." Engaging the powers of the mind with the process of breathing can affect our state of mind for the better. Both Ayurvedic and Chinese medicine use the healing power of breath to bring about remarkable physical cures by restoring balance to body systems.

Conscious breath practices can help to drive away chronic illness. Consciously practiced breath work:

- Helps release uncomfortable feelings or memories.

- Brings more oxygen to the brain and lessens depression.

- Increases mental and physical energy.

- Catalyzes the transformation of nutrients into fuel and improves metabolism.

- Improves the function of internal organs and the immune system.

- Leads to greater insight into self – "Know thyself."

- Connects us with the qualities of soul (love, compassion, joy).

- Minimizes stress and the effects of stress.

# Considerations for Breath Practices

Oxygen is energy. Whenever we breathe in, we breathe in energy. Whenever we breathe out, we expel toxins and tensions, making room for more energy. Sounds made during exhale increase toxin removal. Sounds do not have to be audible, but may be made through internal awareness alone.

Breath may be consciously directed to any place in the body that needs more energy. Placing a hand over a particular organ will help to direct the mind to it: placing a hand over the liver while breathing directly sends energy to the liver.

Be careful not to control the energy. Control and resistance force the energy to express in other ways such as anger, headaches and pain until the resistance gives way. There is no need to be afraid of the energy: the body will learn to integrate it if we do not fight it.

When we change our breathing rhythm we alter our state of consciousness. Restricted breathing limits our capacity for living. Breath follows emotion and changes under the influence of emotion: loving or peaceful feelings manifest in long and easy breaths, sending energy to the heart area; angry breaths come primarily to the upper chest, activating the fight or flight mode; fear makes us hold our breath and contract the abdominal muscles.

# Gentle Breathing Exercises

## The Ah Breath

The "ah breath" is very gentle breath work for two people to practice together. One person lies down on her back. The other watches the rise and fall of her abdomen and begins to gently let out the sound "ah" as the abdomen falls. Do this for about 20 minutes before changing roles. The effect of this on the receiver is that she feels like she is breathing as pure spirit, unencumbered by the heavy processes of the body. This is a very gentle and effective way to bring one to soul-awareness. It is certainly one of the kindest acts one could do for another person.

## Silent Words and Qigong Breathing

Silent, wordless affirmations usually accompany the following gentle breathing practices. Let this time of quiet guide you with insights and inspiration. The following practices are gentle but powerful. Practice morning and evening and any other available time. These two simple practices are suitable for the long-term.

## The Inner Smile Breath

A genuine smile radiates feelings of peace and love.

- While doing this breath practice, consider the breath to be a smile which you can direct to any part of your body. Softening of the eyes with a smile has a direct effect on the autonomic nervous system, helping to bring it into balance. As you breathe in, see your breath as a smile. Direct your smile and breath to your heart, your liver, and other organs. Feel the difference.

- Imagine you are breathing through your heart. How invigorating this is for the heart! Especially if the heart is smiling! In a similar fashion you can breathe through any part of your body or through any particular organ by visualizing the breath happening there.

- Bathe your whole body in breath by breathing through the soles of your feet or hands and directing the energy to your whole body.

There are so many simple things we can do to help ourselves. I encourage everyone to look also beyond the physical for ways to awaken their healing intelligence. This is one exploration that can make illness an avenue for personal growth.

# Taoist Natural Breath and Qigong

According to the Taoists, living in the Tao means living in accord with nature and the universal life force, the highest and best source of healing. This puts us in harmony with the spiritual energies of heaven and the nourishing energies of earth. The Taoists say that a powerful electric field surrounds the planet. Qigong breathing aligns us with this energy field and the motion of the universe. It restores the body to balance and increases vital energy, or *qi*.

Qigong teaches that breathing into the abdomen directs vital energy to and from the *dan tien*, the "elixir field." The *dan tien* is the physical center of gravity located in the abdomen three finger widths below and two finger widths behind the navel. Breathing into the *dan tien* can relieve problems caused by a diaphragm that doesn't move when you breathe. A habit of breathing only into the chest, over time, can be a precipitating factor in many illnesses and a factor in chronic pain. Diaphragmatic breathing to the *dan tien* acts like a pump, pushing *qi* to other parts of the body and improving circulation. When the diaphragm moves freely and the breathing is slow and deep, pain seems to go away and more oxygen goes to the brain, relieving anxiety, excitability, and tension. In China this sort of breathing has been used as a primary treatment for asthma.[87]

Practice abdominal breathing as follows:

1. Imagine the breath staying in the lower abdomen. As you inhale, you expand the *dan tien*. As you exhale, it sinks back.

2. Breathe slowly, deeply, and gently, with long and rhythmic breaths, not forcing it in any way, focusing the mind on the *dan tien* rather than the breath. Mind does not follow the breath—the breath follows the mind.

3. The mind should be calm and empty, not concerned with technique or routine.

4. As the mind settles, so will the breath. Eventually, when the mind and breath settle, the breath will be almost undetectable.[88]

# Professor Saraswati's *Pranayama* for Specific Physical Problems

I present here several breathing methods recommended by Professor Shivananda Saraswati [89] specifically for strengthening a weakened condition or to address certain states of illness. He states that no disease can be perfectly cured without *pranayama* and that *pranayama* is the highest form of medicine. He writes that the practice of *pranayama* alone can eliminate catarrhal diseases including asthma.

## Brahman *Pranayama* (Breathing While Walking) Will Strengthen a Weakened System

Saraswati recommends the following exercises and considers the first one, breathing while walking, to be one of his most miraculous healing breath practices. The exercise is not as complex as it appears: the important thing to remember is that, in this practice, you exhale more air than you take in. If you remember to concentrate on your breathing whenever you go for a walk, this practice is easy to do. Saraswati recommends doing this twice a day, starting at a comfortable level and increasing the number of breaths gradually over time as it becomes easier.

## The practice:

### Beginning:

1. When first starting to practice this exercise, breathe for a total of 6 minutes as you walk.

2. Walking in a place where the air is clean, inhale slowly and steadily with the rhythm of your steps, mentally counting 1, 2, 3, and 4 with each breath.

3. After inhaling fully to this count, exhale to a count of 1, 2, 3, 4, 5, 6, if possible, breathing out more air than you take in. It is also possible to chant "Om" instead of counting.

### Increasing counts:

4. After a few weeks, when the count of 4-in and 6-out becomes easy, increase your walking time to a total of nine minutes. Increase to a 6-in and 8-out count.

### Further increases:

5. Increase the time to a total of 12 minutes. After this gets easy, increase the count to 8 in and 12 out. Once this is mastered, it is not necessary to keep count, just proceed in a rhythmical way.

6. You can gradually increase walking time to a total of 15 minutes.

7. Eventually you can work up to a total walking time of 18 minutes.

As in any endeavor, it is wise to proceed slowly at your own pace with these increases. It is important not to experience any gasping during practice. Once you are able to do this easily for half an hour in the morning and evening, it will provide prophylaxis against diseases that result from weak lungs and will resuscitate a debilitated body. After a couple years of practice, you can do this for an hour at a time.

**A Modern Tool for a Simple Walking and Breath Routine:** If all the counting seems too complicated or demanding, a simple alternative would be to work up to walking 5,000-10,000 steps a day using a pedometer to do the counting for you. 10,000 may be too high a goal for some, but no matter: start where you can. The important part is to remember your breathing and to consciously breathe out more than you breathe in.

## *Pranayama* to Build up the Will and Restore the Whole Body

Lie down in total relaxation, interlocking the fingers over the navel. Inhale deeply through the nose and visualize the "vital force" entering the navel region. Exhale slowly through the nose, visualizing this vital force radiating throughout the nerves, arteries, glands and all the organs, taking away anything that does not need to be there. Do this for three or four minutes to start with.

## *Pranayama* to Bring Vitality to the Blood

Protrude the tip of the tongue through the lips to make it look like a bird's bill; slowly inhale through the tip of the tongue and hold the breath in the throat for five seconds and release the air slowly through the nose. Practice for at least three or four minutes to a maximum of ten minutes. The literature says this will give relief for burning palms and soles and that it is a blood purifier and remedy for skin conditions. The yogis say that this *pranayama*, if practiced faithfully, will bring so much vitality to the blood that one will easily survive being bitten by a venomous snake (or a tick?).

# Energetic Forms of *Pranayama*

The following breath practices are very detoxifying and energizing. They may be performed in sequence. This sequence is especially useful for nerve issues, improved cognition, and depression. This is similar to the protocol followed by Dr. Patricia Gerbarg in overcoming her Lyme disease (with the assistance of the herb rhodiola). Dr. Richard Brown writes that this sort of breathing protocol is helpful in ADHD, heart function, cancer, immune system building, and cognitive functions such as memory and learning.[90] Notable about this practice, besides its benefits for the autonomic nervous system, is that it leads to production of oxytocin, the hormone involved in social bonding, the "cuddle hormone." In major depression oxytocin levels are low.

**Note:** Bellows breath and breath of fire are contraindicated for persons with heart disease, high blood pressure, hiatal hernia, and for pregnant women.

## 1. *Ujjayi* (Victory Breath)

*Ujjayi* is a simple diaphragmatic breath that incorporates a slight constriction in the throat. The aim is to expand first the lower lobes of the lungs, then the middle lobes, then the upper. This sort of slow breathing, airway resistance, breath holding, and expansion of lungs and chest wall has been shown to be restorative for the autonomic nervous system. *Ujjayi* breathing brings energy into the throat and the head.

Dr. Richard Brown summarizes the practice:[91]

1. Slow breathing (2-4 breaths per minute)

2. Contracting of larynx

3. Breathing in with airway resistance

4. Breathing out with airway resistance

5. Holding the breath

**Directions:**

• Sit upright in a comfortable manner.

• Begin by making some sounds like whispering, breathing out words like "hello" through the mouth as you breathe in and out. You will notice that your throat feels somewhat constricted. Think of this as trying to purr like a cat. Maintain the throat restriction on both inhale and exhale.

• Let your awareness rest with the breath as you follow it in and out. Allow your mind to experience the sensations the breath brings with it.

• The action should be from the solar plexus and diaphragm rather than from the chest. The inhale and exhale flow smoothly into each other. If you put your hands around your ribs, thumb towards the back and fingers resting above the hip bone, you can feel the ribs and muscles move as the breath goes in and out.

• Inhale and exhale are of equal duration. The hissing sound should become a continuous sound.

• Do sequences of 11 breaths, resting between each series of 11.

• Gradually lengthen the time of the inhale and exhale.

• Let your awareness rest first with the sensations in the throat and in the navel area. Awareness will soon take you deeper into the mind. When this happens you just go with that.

## 2. *Bhastrika* (Bellows Breath)

**Bhastrika** is a vigorous *pranayama* that clears respiratory obstructions and strengthens the nervous system. It brings energy to both body and mind. The action is in the muscles of the abdomen, which pump the breath in and out like a bellows while the rest of the body remains still.

### Directions:

- Sit upright either in a chair or cross-legged on the floor. If you prefer the floor, sitting on a pillow will help keep the back straight.

- Placing your hands on the abdomen and solar plexus will allow you to feel the muscles pumping and help you to focus on the breath as it brings energy to the area.

- In the beginning, inhalation and exhalation take about 1 second each. Do this for 1-3 rounds. You can hear the breath as you push it vigorously out and pull it back in.

- Increase the pace as you feel able. Focus on the sensations in the breath and body.

- When you start the practice, focus on the navel center. Here again, the focus will eventually move to the eyebrow center and a state of meditation.

Sandra Anderson of the Himalayan Institute recommends the following protocol:[92]

### Beginning daily rounds:

- Start with 1-3 rounds, 7-11 breaths per round, 1 breath per second.

- Rest between rounds.

- Add 5-10 rounds per week as lung capacity increases.

- Gradually increase to 2 breaths per second.

- You may eventually increase the total time.

## 3. *Om* Chant

After *bhastrika*, chant the mantra "Om" three times as you exhale. Exhales here are long and slow with a 15 second rest between each chant.

A mantra is a phrase or word that has the power to bring spiritual benefits to the speaker. Mantras come from deep consciousness rather than from the intellect. As practiced by the ancient rishis a mantra could condense into one or more syllables even a long treatise of several thousand verses. "*Om*" is the universal sound which activates the psychic centers. It is considered the most powerful of sounds, for it incorporates the energy of the universe and encompasses all knowledge on all planes of being. Ancient scriptures say that using this mantra alone can bring enlightenment. According to Joachim-Ernst Berendt,

> If you say *OM* in the correct way, leading the sound from the head through the chest down into the belly, then the entire body will start to vibrate. The M in particular, spoken forcefully, can make the body vibrate for a long time. In fact the body will continue to vibrate when the mantra (beginning again with the O) is "threaded" into the head once more and led down again. At that point not only the chest, stomach, and belly will be vibrating, but also the head and (if you have practiced enough) even your arms and legs.[93]

## 4. *Kapalabhati* (Breath of Fire)

Breath of fire is very energetic. It creates heat in the body, cleans the blood, and supports the nervous system. It takes some effort to learn it, as it does not come naturally. It is best to do this practice under medical advisement, or at least with modification to accommodate individual needs and capabilities. As a cleansing breath it enhances elimination of metabolic wastes, carbon dioxide, and mucus congestion.

- Find a stable sitting posture.

- If you bring your hands to your belly without pressing on it, you can feel the abdomen contracting sharply on exhalation, rebounding without effort on inhalation. Exhalation is forceful, whereas inhalation is passive and effortless. It is important to quickly relax after the exhalation.

- There should be no movement anywhere except in the abdomen. You may need to raise the arms over the head to the back of the shoulders to help keep the chest out of the action.

- Start with 1 breath every couple seconds for a total of 7-11 breaths.

- Rest.

- Do another round of 7-11 breaths.

As always, the mental focus is on the breath and inner sensations. When you begin, focus on the navel center and then let your attention eventually rest on the eyebrow center.

Sandra Anderson recommends the following sequences:[94]

### Beginning this practice:

- 1-3 rounds of 7-11 breaths, 1 breath per second.

- Rest between rounds.

- Add 5-10 breaths per round each week.

- Gradually pick up speed to 2 breaths per second.

- Work up to 3 or more minutes at this speed.

Do not jump into a full, energetic practice of breath of fire before sufficient lung capacity has developed. Always begin these practices at a comfortable pace.

Though I have placed this chapter at the end of the book, breath practices should not be discounted: they could possibly be the most invigorating and healing of all the protocols. Breathwork practices combine well with the next chapter, "Spirit."

# TWELVE

# Spirit

*You are not a drop in the ocean.*
*You are the entire ocean, in a drop.*

Rumi

**Rapture:** *Music in the soul can be heard by the universe.*

Lao Tsu

## Holographic Healing

We have within us an infinite source of beauty. This beauty is the cradle of true healing, the creative power of the mind to create and restore. Accessing this source of beauty keeps the sometimes destructive influence of the external world subdued and in its place. By consciously engaging this source of beauty, we open ourselves to increased learning abilities, greater intuition, improved focus, greater concentration, and greatly increased personal self-awareness. These states of mind are the source of dreaming and the ability to create holographically and spontaneously.

Meditative states bring the brain into a state of union with great mysteries, and influence the calming, restorative parasympathetic nervous system. Deep meditative states resonate at the same frequency as the earth. They give us the strength of the earth, bringing heart and mind together. When heart and mind come together we can more easily and spontaneously flow, adapt to change, and deal with obstacles.

Deeper brain frequencies radiate waves of healing energy. This is life uniting with itself. Meditative practices (spirit) draw energy into the body, for according to Taoist theory, energy follows spirit, allowing spirit to command energy. This stops energy from leaking out through the senses and the emotions. It also benefits the physical body, for it links the mind with the immune system.[95] The Taoists believe that restoration of *shen* (spirit) leads to perfection of consciousness and awareness of the illusions of the senses. Seeking the return of *shen* is the essence of all human life and existence. They teach that without spirit, we die.[96] It goes without saying that any form of meditation is beneficial for the spirit. Practiced over time it has the power to change brain chemistry and structure.

A regular practice of some sort of meditative absorption will strengthen the deeper powers of the mind and the will. We are capable of different things in the different mind states. The tools for accessing the higher states are almost limitless: *pranayama*, drumming, story, meditation, music, and poetry are only a few of the ways we can begin to do this. Following are some characteristics of the various brain frequencies:

| Frequency | Effect |
|---|---|
| Delta (1-4 Hz) | Deep dreamless sleep |
| | Lucid dreaming |
| | Problem-solving |
| | Immune system repair |
| | Collective unconscious |

| | |
|---|---|
| Theta (4-8 Hz) | Waking dream, dream-like imagery |
| | Healing trauma through dreams |
| | The unconscious |
| | Recall of ancient memory |
| | Holistic think-ing, inspiration |
| | Visualization and free association |
| | Shamanic journeys |
| | Creativity, in-sight, intuition |
| Schumann resonance (7.8 Hz) | Resonance of the earth |
| | Can be achieved dur-ing meditation |
| Alpha (8-12 Hz) | Nonlinear think-ing, inner-directed |
| | "Twilight" state just before sleep |
| | Deep relaxation |
| | Receptive to learning |
| | Mood elevation |
| | Emotional balance |

| | |
|---|---|
| Beta (13-21 Hz) | Wide awake, dealing with normal events<br>Thinking<br>Sustained attention, focus<br>Associated with anxiety and tension |
| High beta (20-32 Hz) | Intense alertness<br>Kundalini, tantra<br>Subject to anxiety |
| Gamma (38-42 Hz) | Brain works holographically<br>Higher consciousness<br>Compassion, altruism |

# Music and Binaural Beat Technology

For those who are unable to sit still long enough to meditate, modern technology, itself a product of exceedingly active brains, has provided brain wave entrainment (BWE) methods to help slow our restless brain frequencies. "Entrainment" refers to the synchronization of two or more rhythmic cycles to form a unified beat. The remarkable effect of brainwave entrainment is that it puts the listener very quickly into a deep state of meditation where the mind becomes deeply creative. People in this state feel like this is "home."

Deeper states may be accessed very quickly through binaural beat music or sounds. Binaural beat music is engineered to have a slight variation in the frequencies heard in the right and left ears: one sound is pulsed into the left ear and a slightly different sound is pulsed into the right ear. This will cause the brain to generate and hear a third sound that is not audible to the ears, which is equivalent to the difference between the two pulses coming into each ear. This is the binaural beat. You can hear it when the right hemisphere of the brain is acting in unison with the left hemisphere. This is the beat your brainwaves will entrain to. It stresses the brain slightly, making it attempt to grow neural pathways and produce endorphins. Earphones are required in order to get this effect when listening to binaural music.

Brain wave entrainment improves brain metabolism (neurotransmitters) as well as cerebral blood flow, leading to improvement in conditions such as obsessive-compulsive disorder (OCD), attention deficit/hyperactivity disorder (ADHD), depression,[97] and anxiety.[98] BWE provides an effective treatment for seasonal affective disorder (SAD) and other conditions.[99]

One of my favorite binaural CDs is "Winds over the World" from Hemi-Sync (Monroe Institute) by J. S. Epperson, although many others are available. Smart phone technology makes it easy to bring all this to your time of falling asleep. Other MP3 binaural beat music may be downloaded to computer or smart phone from Amazon cloud.

## Get Your Beauty Sleep

Music has the power to change your life. The healing qualities of music are not limited to binaural beat technology. Music that moves your spirit can take you to deep, healing states. Listening to healing music is a practice of choice for calming the system and creating more positive mind states. I believe that disease states become less aggressive when flooded with peaceful sounds.

Put on earphones and listen to peaceful music, either regular or binaural beat music, just before going to sleep. Put your left hand over your heart and your right hand over your solar plexus. Close your eyes and, as you listen to the music, let your eyes focus straight ahead through the eyebrow center into the darkness, looking to see what it reveals. The only thing you need to do is to relinquish any thoughts left over from the day, or any worries about the future. You may see colors as you feel your attention becoming, of its own accord, more focused and less desirous of trying to figure anything out.

This is a good time to let your affirmations, your heart's desires, and your intentions for healing reveal themselves. In this self-created state there is no need for lengthy scripts. Your inner healer will do the talking for you and will teach you to direct the energies created in these states to those parts of you that most need healing.

If you get in the habit of doing this every night it will not be long before you notice your dreams becoming much more colorful and alive; inspiration will come to you about what you need to do next in your life. Practiced over time this can be an antidote to worry and anxiety. It can restore you to all that is good about being human. Most of all, it will bring harmony to the cells of your body and your immune system. The possibilities are infinite.

# The Power of Inspiring Words

*The subconscious law of success is to repeat affirmations*
*intensely and attentively immediately before sleep and after sleep.*
*Doubt not; when you want to obtain any righteous goal,*
*cast away the thought of failure.*

## Self-Talk

Barbara Hoberman Levine healed herself of cancer by becoming acutely aware of how speech affects our ability to heal. Her book *Your Body Believes Every Word* You Say spells out in a non-judgmental, non-shaming way how to substitute positive words for those negative words that sabotage any healing process. I quote from *Total Healing to the Limits:*[100]

...We find in our own everyday habits the repetition *ad infinitum* of punishing words. . . Levine writes that our body hears these words in a very literal and honest way, believing that these words are true. It then obliges us by performing as the words dictate. By doing our best to root out these mindlessly repeated attacks upon ourselves, we take responsibility for our own health. Levine suggests avoiding destructive expressions such as the following:

"It blows my mind"

"I'm losing my nerve"

"It makes me crazy"

"I feel terrible"

"I'm sick and tired"

"Heartbroken"

With a little effort, we can observe how easily we use negative suggestion. We can then create for ourselves a vocabulary that expresses our own strength in a positive, energetic way.

## Affirmations

Positive self-affirmation is a simple process to learn, however certain steps need to be carefully followed. The first step is to determine exactly what you wish to accomplish. Then form a mental image or feeling associated with that. This is a good time to use any metaphors or images you have come up with about your illness or issues. See yourself in a desired situation or create a picture of a desired outcome. Let your mind return to this image frequently with positive energy. If you're aware of a negative statement that you keep repeating to yourself, try rephrasing this in a positive way and use this as your visualization statement. The general format for visualizations described by Shakti Gawain is as follows:[101]

- The first word of an affirmation is usually "I."

- Avoid words that suggest doubt, such as "maybe," "probably," "try," or "if."

- Always use the present tense "I am . . ." It is happening NOW.

- Use positive words because the unconscious rejects negatives like "less," "not," "don't," or "won't."

- Be affirmative because the unconscious mind welcomes that.

- Know that you will succeed. Know that you will do whatever it takes to make it happen. Self-help is about helping ourselves rather than expecting someone else to do it for us.

- Use mental images. The unconscious thinks in images and metaphors. The altered state will easily suggest images for you. Every single one of is an artist.

- Work with only one suggestion at a time.

## Affirmations Larger-Than-Life

An interesting variation on affirmations, especially when done in the theta state is to add the word "command" to the statement. This can lead to a real sense of personal power over one's situation as well as an almost tangible sense that your commands are directly affecting the restoration of balance to the natural workings of body systems. Bearing in mind the suggestions above to use a positive mindset and deliberate avoidance of negative words, one might elaborate on commands such as:[102]

> I command my bloodstream to gently neutralize any unwelcome bacteria and to restore balance to my system, NOW!
>
> I command resolution to my issues of loneliness, NOW!
>
> I command a healing for my (depression, liver, neuropathy, etc.) NOW!
>
> I command all my spiritual gifts be brought forth, with ease, into my conscious awareness, bringing with them wisdom

and understanding, NOW!

I command all my issues related to my feelings of victimization be released, NOW!

I command the genes causing my disease be identified and replaced with genes providing me with perfect health, NOW!

I command my body be returned to its perfect state of wholeness, NOW!

I command my creativity to bring forth new inspiration to further my self-healing wisdom, NOW!

I command any damaged organ systems be restored to a state of perfect health, NOW!

I command any toxic debris be released from my body gently and with ease, NOW!

I command my inner wisdom to seek out only health-giving foods and non-harmful healing methods, NOW!

# Self-Hypnosis

Self-created affirmations and visualizations are much more powerful when practiced in deeper states of consciousness. While you are in a higher mind state (theta state) allow your mind's eye to see images of yourself healing or spirochetes going away or your immune system becoming strong. These images do not need to be aggressive. Peaceful images work very well.

The power of words thus repeated, perhaps in tandem with binaural beat meditation, has the power to initiate change in your body. These periods of greater suggestibility may be used to introduce positive energy for healing through auto-suggestion, repeating phrases which change negative, unworkable beliefs into positive thoughts. Affirmations combined with visualizations in the alpha or theta states are the best way to initiate change in attitude and will.

Some may choose to work with consciously practiced self-hypnosis for these times of self-healing. Self-hypnosis is an extended form of positive affirmation that uses scripts designed for particular purposes. Though self-hypnosis is beyond the scope of this book, it is worth looking into for the serious self-healer. You may buy guided self-hypnosis visualization CDs or you can record your own scripts.

## Incorporating Gratitude

We can ease ourselves out of an unhappy state if we learn to incorporate gratitude into our self-statements. Gratitude is a primary tool for spiritual wellness. It also sends healing to the body. Thoughts of gratitude are life-enhancing. Use phrases that begin with "I am . . ." and "I have . . ." instead of "I want . . ."

- I am grateful for everything I have received, including this opportunity to learn to heal myself.

- I am happy that I am getting better.

- I visualize myself as whole, healthy, and happy.

- I am grateful and happy to have all the support I need.

# THIRTEEN

# A Workable Program

*The world is full of suffering;*
*it is full also of the overcoming of it.*

Helen Keller

Starting a healing program may look like a hopelessly complex task. In reality, it is necessary only to start with one simple thing. Anything you do can inspire and lead to a next step or a new outlook. The energy has a will to be, a will to spring into existence, to move through stagnation to create something new.

It helps to have a basic understanding of what is going on with you so that you can look for remedies. You need to have a clear, basic picture of:

- How your body defends itself and what it needs in order to do that

- Whatever habits are causing or exacerbating your condition

- What you can do to fortify your inner strength and determination

## A Philosophy for Constructing a Program

It helps to articulate your goals and what you are willing to do to achieve them. It will probably look different for each person. I offer my philosophy as an example:

1. It has to be inexpensive enough that I can afford to do it for as long as it takes.

2. I like to incorporate freely-available natural herbs such as fresh burdock root or fresh nettles and other herbs in season. Tinctures and teas are easy to make.

3. It has to involve mega-nutrition through fresh vegetable juices and a high energy diet.

4. It has to be easy enough to do so I can follow it every day. It has to be non-stressful, non-disgusting, and non-heroic, as well as affordable. It must be do-able in terms of energy expenditure and ease of carrying it through.

5. I am also willing to commit to brief periods of heroic therapies if necessary, though that is getting harder and harder to even consider.

6. I should be able to fit most of it into a dedicated hour first thing in the morning or any other time that fits my schedule.

7. It has to be simple, though I prefer to have a basic understanding of what makes it work.

8. Whatever I do must be as close to natural as possible because I do not want to be left with possible life-long side-effects.

9. I want to be able to directly feel the effects from most of what I do or take, or to at least have enough faith in what I am doing to make me believe it is working. I need to learn to distinguish between a Herxheimer reaction and a flare-up so I don't stop anything too soon.

10. I need a positive thumbs-up from intuition informed by sufficient research, to validate whatever I am doing.

11. Ideally, it should make me feel good, energized, and posi-

tive: at the least it should contribute to assisting me to accept, receive, and believe in my own reality. Feeling good helps us to handily create positive self-statements.

12. I need to keep the daily supplement list to a manageable quantity of pills to take every day. I have to take the right supplements for particular needs (which may change from day to day).

13. I need to bring beauty into the healing process. This would be anything that brings me to creativity, intuition, and wisdom.

## Step by Step: Cultivating Personal Habits

Where would someone start? Of necessity, we must first answer the cries of the physical body for healing. It could be overwhelming to try to do everything at once, so it is important to find your comfort level and adjust it over time. A person could start anywhere, but should bear in mind that the first four points are fundamental to all the rest.

1. Eliminate foods that harm your immune system and feed your invaders.

2. Support yourself with life-giving foods, particularly juices and green smoothies. Restore your methylation cycle (immune system) with proper supplements and foods. Devise a diet that works for you. Alkalize!

3. Support your liver and your digestive processes; restore intestinal flora.

4. Take in more oxygen to increase energy levels and boost important body processes. This can be through exercise, perhaps walking or swimming; or Professor Saraswati's walking and breathing routine; or breath work and *pranayama*; or yoga and qigong. Ozone is also a therapy of choice here.

5. Jumpstart your program with regular heat therapies to improve any mood problems and to provide "heat shock" proteins to stimulate the immune system and deal with flare-ups.

6. Consult a naturopath knowledgeable about Lyme and chronic fatigue.

7. Decide whether you need to purchase equipment such as an ozone generator, infrared sauna, rebounder, juicer, or blender.

8. Harmonize your brain and your cells with beautiful music and meditative practices. Start with some binaural beat music. Go into this space every night before sleep.

9. You may want to practice healing affirmations or self-hypnosis. Learn to substitute positive imagery and words for negative, self-destructive images and words.

10. Do web searches and other research to see what others have done to heal themselves from your disease. Doctors do not have the time to give you everything you need.

If flare-ups threaten, I always come back to my simple program:

- Green juices and smoothies (which I should never have stopped doing) to lessen acidity in the body and give me strength.

- Diligence in following a dedicated ozone protocol and whatever supplements make the most sense to me at the time, particularly antimicrobials and adaptogens.

- And I remember to take them.

- I make sure I keep practicing conscious relaxation and meditation to stay in touch with the inner healer.

## A Simplified Diet for Healing

Perhaps your intestinal function has been wrecked by sugar and antibiotics. The most important thing you can do to get back on track is to adopt a diet that will rebuild your system and banish weird symptoms. Changing eating habits takes thought and determination. It can take a couple years to get it the way you want it. But it is a worthwhile thing to do.

For people recovering from an illness it would seem that some combination of a living food diet, the Paleolithic diet, and the Gerson diet would be ideal for the self-healer. The aim is to reduce acidity in the body, to thin mucus and reduce lymph swelling, to energize, and to create peaceful states of consciousness. This diet would consist of:

- Lots of raw, organically grown vegetables and a moderate amount of fruit

- Green juices and smoothies, possibly fortified with superfoods such as spirulina

- Fermented foods and high-fiber foods such as chia and other seeds

- Avoidance of grains, beans, cheese, and processed foods designed in a laboratory

- Emphasis on foods high in glutathione and phytosterols

- Only pasture-raised lean meat (if you eat meat at all)

- Only free-rage chicken and eggs. "Cage free" is not free range.

- Only olive oil and coconut oil to be used as oils

# 9 Popular Ways to Subvert Healing Efforts

Nobody is perfect, they say. We all slip up now and then. It is important that we not scold ourselves or feel bad when this happens.

We just climb back on and resume our program. We may get derailed if we:

1. Eat sugar and allergenic foods.

2. Hang out with negative, discouraging people.

3. Have poor sleeping habits or not enough sleep.

4. Neglect making time for meditative or breathwork practices.

5. Indulge in depressive thoughts, self-hatred, worry and catastrophic thinking.

6. Neglect getting enough exercise.

7. Procrastinate, put off getting started, or never get around to doing what we need to do.

8. Let unforeseen events or financial worries derail our good intentions.

9. Watching too much TV (this constitutes a wholly different mindset).

Restoring health through natural self-healing is a long process. I cannot stress enough that it takes dedication. This much you can count on: if this is where your concentration lies, your dreams at night will help you know what to do.

## Away from Home

If you have to be away from home for a week or longer it is tempting to just hope for the best and not put too much thought into maintaining whatever regimens you are on. However, to avoid becoming sick in a place where you may not be eating properly or may not have access to resources, it is imperative to take along whatever supplements will help keep you from backtracking or getting sick.

The following is a list of things I took on a recent trip. I packed the supplements into labeled sandwich bags and kept them at the dinner table so I would not forget to take them. This list was appropriate for me at the time: it might vary at other times. The critical idea is to list a few supplements you most need for immune support or antimicrobial support and take them with you when you go. In the future I would be sure to include essential oils in my list. When I was away I was able to begin every day with whole lemon drink with garlic, olive oil, and parsley. I tried to have at least some fresh juice every day. I took along:

> Reishi mushrooms for immune support
>
> Vitamin C (buffered)
>
> B vitamins
>
> Resveratrol/Japanese knotweed for Lyme
>
> Curcumin for everything
>
> Garlic tablets for everything
>
> Rhodiola and eleuthero for adrenal support and energy
>
> Oregon grape root just in case I got sick (antimicrobial)
>
> Artemesinin, in case of a babesia flareup
>
> Magnesium oil in case of muscle spasms
>
> Melatonin and honokiol for sleep

## Putting it Together

Below is a rough list of things I consider worth doing every day. The list may change from time to time as conditions change. The only caution is the basic rule of not letting ozone cancel out supplements or food: wait at least 15 minutes after doing ozone; wait 6 hours after Vitamin C or other antioxidant to do ozone. Also, it is best to do the most energizing practices early in the day. This would include the adaptogens, vitamin C flushes, EWOT, etc. This is a demanding list, but over time it becomes easier to maintain the discipline it calls for.

# Example of an Everyday Program

## Early Morning Long-Term Program

1. Ozone, ozonated water, ozone saunas and/or insufflations to kill spirochetes, support immune system, and enhance energy. Consistent use can provide great relief or healing.

2. Systemic enzymes taken before eating anything and after doing ozone, for removal of blood clots, biofilms, and neurotoxins.

3. Essential oils in the morning. Use oils appropriate for antibiotic purposes, particular symptoms, or reducing biofilms. These are reported to be extremely effective for Lyme.

4. Whole lemon drink (with garlic) for lymphatic congestion, liver flushing, immune support, and help with neuropathies.

5. If you are doing infrared saunas it helps to do this after these other things. We tend to forget this sort of thing as we get involved with our daily life.

## Morning or Any Time

1. Breakfast on vegetable juices, green smoothies or wheatgrass juice for energy and deep cellular healing. This helps keep things from getting worse. Greens support inner strength and wellbeing, enhanced immune function, energy, and inner cleansing.

2. *Pranayama* or EWOT (exercise with oxygen) for circulation, rejuvenation, improved blood flow and transport of oxygen. This practice can lead to improved mood, good feelings, and inner strength.

3. Heat (saunas, FIR saunas, hot tubs, ozone saunas) for improved circulation, lymphatic flow, and for relief from symptoms. Heat shock is a major support for the immune system.

4. Glutathione precursors such as B12 shots or other supplements for support of the methylation cycle. This is a crucial link in the immune processes as well a primary tool for restoring brain function and improving mood.

5. Adaptogens such as rhodiola, eleuthero, or green tea for adrenal stimulation, fortification against disease, general coping strength, improved sense of well-being and increased energy.

6. Magnesium supplementation to replace magnesium depleted by spirochetes and to help with depression and muscle spasms.

# Before Bed

1. LDN (low-dose naltrexone) for immune stimulation. Side-effects are a more active dream life and improved mood.

2. For good sleep try melatonin or honokiol (magnolia bark). Good sleep is vital for recovery and maintaining energy for the next day.

3. Meditation, breath work, binaural beat music, self-hypnosis, or qigong. Although these can be practiced any time for stress reduction and inner healing, they are particularly helpful before bed to create more peaceful sleep.

# Any Time

1. Extra virgin coconut oil, taken with food, is very powerful for a variety of symptoms and as a brain food. It is effective

against candida and viruses and it can lead to a dramatic decrease in neurological symptoms.

2. Exercise and sunlight keep the lymph flowing and help sustain energy. Exercise has a synergistic effect with everything else you might do. It also helps decrease anxiety and improve mood.

3. Supplements as needed for daily maintenance, immune support, and health restoration.

# Some Final Observations about Natural Healing

I will leave you with some small truths that will offer encouragement for staying on the path:

- Nature has answers for us. Nature gave us this disease and nature is merciful enough to provide the tools we need if we can work cooperatively with it. Nature has a healing program for us if we can learn to listen for it. Antibiotics do not work with nature.

- Cooperate with nature rather than fight it. Killing spirochetes is not the answer. Making ourselves strong is the answer.

- Nature will support anyone who has the determination and the desire to heal.

- We do have the intention and the discipline to carry out long-term measures. We do have the fortitude to stay with it and not give in to impulses that would derail our healing efforts. For the long term, gentle and steady wins the race.

- We can't talk our way out of this. This illness demands our attention. There is no avoiding its insistent calls for us to understand it and do something about it. We simply have to deal with it.

- Healing calls for life-style adjustments. Life as we have always known it has to change, not because it was bad, but because many of our former activities can undermine our health. This is particularly evident in the area of social life and the prevalence of addictive treats. We have to revise our eating habits: No more bread, cookies, cheesecake, wine, soft drinks, and beer. Wah! But it eventually gets easier as we realize we are gaining control over the illness.

- Illness changes us in good ways. There is no doubt that serious illness can change our life in dramatic ways. The transformed being that we have become may not look like anything we ever imagined for ourselves. We can become so changed that we no longer fit into old frameworks or social concepts. We can choose to see ourselves either as smaller or as larger. We become explorers venturing with trepidation and curiosity into unfamiliar but attractive territory. The journey reveals more to us about life than we could ever imagine. If we welcome and value the deeper connection with ourselves that illness brings, we will realize that the ultimate tool for healing lies within ourselves, and that we will end up healing parts of ourselves we never thought needed healing.

# Appendix A

## Life-Friendly Recipes

*Bear in mind that you should conduct yourself in life as at a feast.*

Epictetus

**Delight**: "Delectation, feast, joy, manna, pleasure, treat."

Merriam-Webster Dictionary

The recipes below are included for their healing properties, not necessarily for culinary artistry. Some of the suggested recipes may initially bring on cleansing reactions. If this happens, limit intake or adjust the quantity of ingredients until the body can adapt. Over time the body will learn to welcome foods with strong healing properties. Dietary changes should be approached with common sense. There is no need to be overly heroic in this. Transitions from a poor diet can take up to a couple years. Or they may occasionally happen overnight.

### Formula for Protein Shakes or Smoothies

Protein shakes are a combination of two or more ingredients blended until smooth. If you use isolated whey protein powder do not add fruit, since fruit degrades it. A basic recipe for protein smoothies can have a base such as:

- A banana, blended fruit, sunflower or sesame milk, raw tahini milk, or coconut milk

- Left-over sesame, sunflower or almond mush from making seed milks

- Protein powder such as hemp or pumpkin seed (sugar-free)

- Rejuvelac or raw apple juice for thinning the mixture

**Optional:**

- Carob powder or spices such as cinnamon

- Soaked, dried figs, prunes, dates or raisins for extra sweetener

- Nuts and seeds

- Alfalfa or other sprouts

# Fermented Foods

Fermented foods made at home are far superior in supplying friendly bacteria for healing the gut than any supplemental probiotic on the market. Fermentation is a living enzyme process, quite different from the process of rotting, which involves decomposition (not a desirable diet!).

# Rejuvelac

Rejuvelac provides *lactobacillus* for healing the gut and aiding digestion. Well-made rejuvelac tastes like lemonade. If it tastes bad, throw it out. You can start by drinking a glass a day and building up from there. Use rejuvelac instead of water when making sauces or smoothies.

**Tools Needed:**

Wide-mouth gallon jar for soaking wheat berries

Screening or cheese cloth to cover, with rubber band

Blender or food processor

Sprout bag or cheesecloth for draining sprouted wheat

Distilled water

1. Soak ½ cup of any kind of organic wheat berries overnight. Some prefer the soft white berries. Cover the jar with screening or cheesecloth held in place by a rubber band.

2. Let stand overnight and drain it the next morning. Make sure the jar is tilted so that air still gets in (without air the sprouts would rot)

3. Continue sprouting the berries by rinsing and draining them twice a day for two more days.

4. Place the sprouted berries in a blender with 4 or more cups of distilled water. Wheat berries should be chopped just enough to break them open and no more.

5. Place the chopped berries in a half-gallon jar and fill with water.

6. Let them sit for another two days, stirring a couple times a day.

7. Strain through a sprout bag and place in jars for storage in the refrigerator.

The used berries may be fermented one more time: cover them with water again and let them sit until done. The second batch will ferment faster than the first batch did.

Drink rejuvelac throughout the day.

## Fermented Vegetables

**Note:** to any of the following recipes you may add other peeled vegetables of choice such as squash, carrots, sweet potatoes, dill, and various greens. For more mineral content, add sea vegetables such as dulse and presoaked wakame, arame or hijiki. Fermenting time is about 4 days in the summer and up to 7 days in winter. The batch is done when the flavor is just right. The longer it ferments, the stronger the taste will become. The fermentation process is anaerobic, so it is important to make sure there are no air pockets in the mix.

## Tools needed:

Food processor for chopping vegetables

Small earthen-ware crock pot or other suitable vessel

Tool for pounding sauerkraut: kraut-pounder or other suitable instrument. If you are making large quantities you may want to use a baseball bat. It is possible to buy a small kraut pounder for small batches, but there is usually something lying around the house that will do the job.

Distilled water

Cheesecloth

Plate to cover mixture

Weight to put on plate

## Four Day Sauerkraut

1 head of red or green cabbage, finely shredded in food processor

½ tsp. of caraway seeds and/or celery seeds and/or dill seeds, if desired

1 tsp. of kelp

Several loose cabbage leaves

**Optional:** Layer thinly sliced or shredded beets or other vegetable with the cabbage.

1. Pound the cabbage to bring out the juice and eliminate air pockets.

2. Place vegetables in a small crock or Mason jar; cover with distilled water.

3. Spread the outer leaves of the cabbage on top of the mixture to keep the air out.

4. Place a plate on top of the mixture and put a weight such as a brick or a jug of water on it.

5. Cover with cheesecloth or other cloth.

6. It will be ready any time after 4 days.

7. Scoop off any mold from the top, place the sauerkraut in jars, and refrigerate. Mold will appear only on areas that have been exposed to air. The anaerobic fermentation process is totally safe if the vegetables have been adequately covered with cabbage leaves and protected from air.

## Fermented Beets

Follow the procedure for four-day sauerkraut, using very thinly sliced or shredded beets instead of cabbage.

1. Layer the beets in a small crock with sliced red onions if desired.

2. Cover with distilled water.

3. Cover with cabbage leaves and a weight.

4. Place a cloth over the crock and let stand for four days.

5. Remove the cabbage leaves.

6. Skim off mold and refrigerate.

## Fermented Cabbage Juice

This cabbage drink is a remedy for constipation.

> 1 green or red cabbage, keep outer leaves
>
> Distilled water

1. Chop cabbage in a food processor or blender.
2. Add distilled water and blend the cabbage more.
3. Pour it in a crock, cover well with distilled water.
4. Cover the blended cabbage with outer cabbage leaves or paper towels.
5. Let it stand at room temperature for 3 days.
6. Strain the mixture through a sprout bag or strainer.
7. Discard the pulp and store the juice in a jar in the refrigerator. Note: the pulp is quite smelly and should be removed from the house immediately.

When making further batches, add a cup of the juice from the first batch to the new batch to shorten the fermenting time. Cover the second batch with cabbage leaves, let sit for a day, strain, and refrigerate.

Drink about ½ cup of this three times a day. The juice will keep up to 24 hours in the refrigerator.

## Fermented Beet Juice

> Raw beets
>
> Distilled or filtered water

1. Chop beets in food processor.
2. Add water and blend slightly.
3. Pour into a crock and cover well with distilled water.

4. Cover with cabbage leaves if you have them, or paper towels.

5. Let the mixture stand unrefrigerated for 3 days.

6. Strain the mixture through a sprout bag or fine strainer.

7. Store the juice in a jar in the refrigerator.

The initial batch may be used to start another batch. Fermented beet juice keeps well for a few weeks in the refrigerator.

# Sprouted Seed Foods

Sprouted seeds and nuts are excellent sources of easily digested protein. They are either predigested by the sprouting process or carry their own enzymes. Sunflower seed paté, raw tahini, and seed milks are good staple foods.

All sprouted seeds contain many times more enzymes and phytosterols than the unsprouted seeds. Sprouted alfalfa, mung beans, and other seeds are considered juicy vegetables. Broccoli sprouts are considerably more potent than the mature plant. Seeds of red clover, a blood cleanser and a source of phytoestrogens, make a good addition to other sprout mixtures. Many exotic mixes are available commercially. Sprout fenugreek seeds with alfalfa to create a great lymph stimulator.

Eat sprouted greens in salads, add to raw soups, or juice with other vegetables.

Most raw food recipe books have tables for sprouting all sorts of other seeds, as well as recipes for such things as hummus made with sprouted garbanzos. Automatic sprouters are nice to have, though the old fashioned way of sprouting in jars and rinsing the sprouts works quite well.

## How to Sprout Seeds

Use a wide-mouth quart jar, gallon jug, or nylon sprout bag. If you can find wide-mouth plastic jugs with handles, sprouting is easier.

Use a piece of plastic screening and a rubber band to cover the top of the jar, or use special lids obtainable from health food stores.

1. Thinly cover the bottom of the jar with a layer of seeds.

2. Cover well with water and soak 4-6 hours. If using a sprout bag, soak it overnight in a pan and hang it up to drain in the morning.

3. Drain the water. Be sure to rest the jar at an angle to let some air in so the sprouts do not die and rot.

4. Let the jar drain until next rinsing.

5. Rinse a couple times a day by covering the sprouts with water and draining.

6. Sprouts will be ready in four to six days.

7. Take them out of the jar and spread them on a tray, cover the tray with plastic and put near a window out of direct sunlight for a day to let them become greener. A garden flat with a plastic dome cover works well for this.

8. When the sprouts are green enough, wash them in a large pan or bucket of water, swishing them around to remove the old seed hulls. The spent hulls rot quickly: removing them will allow the sprouts to keep longer.

9. Lift the new sprouts out of the water and place them in a strainer.

10. When sprouts have drained enough, place them in a container and refrigerate them. They will keep for a few days to a week if they are rinsed and drained regularly.

Sprout mung bean and adzuki beans in the usual way until their tails are the length of the seed or a little longer. These are delicious sprinkled over salads or other dishes.

To grow mung beans with long tails, you need to sprout them in darkness under some pressure. Pressure causes the sprout to grow longer to overcome the poor light. For small quantities, a clay terracotta flowerpot works well. Cover the hole in the bottom of the pot with screening and/or a wet paper towel to keep the roots from escaping or drying out.

1. Soak mung beans overnight, and then drain well.

2. Cover the bottom of the pot with one layer of the soaked beans. Cover the pot with a saucer to keep light out.

3. Rinse two or three times a day in running water for a couple minutes.

4. When the sprouts are a few days old, put a small plate right on top of them. Put a weight such as a small stone on the plate.

5. Keep rinsing the sprouts well until they are ready. Inadequate rinsing is the main cause of mung sprout failures.

6. Refrigerate and rinse regularly.

# Seed Milks

Sprouted raw almond, sesame, and sunflower seed milks are good milk substitutes and rich sources of phytosterols. I once made cantaloupe seed milk, and it was the best of all!

**Tools Needed:**

Blender or coffee mill for grinding seeds

Distilled water or water filter to ensure nontoxic water

Nylon sprout bags for straining seed milks

Jar for sprouting

**Handy gadget:** Soy milk machine for making rice, sesame,

sunflower, and nut milks. The machine you buy should be capable of functioning in cold mode. Though I do not recommend using soy in any form, the soy milk machine is a great time-saver for making other seed milks. If you are using a soy milk machine fill it to the water mark with filtered water and soak the seeds overnight in the small strainer in the machine itself. Seed milks should always be processed with the machine in cold mode.

## Seed Milks

Cover 1 cup of seeds with 2 or more cups of filtered water or rejuvelac.

1. Soak overnight.

2. Blend seeds and water thoroughly and press through a tough sprout/strainer bag.

**Optional:** add cinnamon, vanilla, carob, cacao or other flavoring. For added sweetener blend in a few soaked dates.

Sesame milk may also be made by blending raw tahini from a natural food store with filtered water to desired taste.

## Almond Milk

**Note:** raw almonds have disappeared from stores except for some alternative natural food stores. Most available almonds have been pasteurized. Raw almonds need to be ordered from small growers or from Azure Standard.

1. Soak 1 or more cups of raw almonds overnight.

2. Blend with 6 cups of filtered water and strain.

Almond milk may be sweetened by blending in a few soaked dates. It may also be made by blending 2 Tbsp. of raw almond butter in 1 cup of water. Almond cream left over from making almond milk makes a delicious topping for fruit salads and pies.

# To Make Raw Tahini

1 cup raw, untoasted sesame seeds, sprouted and drained twice a day for 2 days

1 tsp. sesame oil

½ tsp. kelp powder (optional)

2 cups warm water.

1. Put sprouted seeds and water in Vitamix or other powerful blender and blend until smooth, adding a little more water if necessary.

2. Put tahini in airtight container. It will keep in the refrigerator for about 3 days.

## Sunflower Pâté

Sunflower pâté is a good staple protein food. It forms a basis for many dishes such as salad dressings and spreads. Most people use Bragg liquid aminos instead of kelp, but if you are avoiding salt, the kelp is preferable.

2 cups raw, shelled sunflower seeds

Juice of 1 or more lemons

1 Tbsp. kelp powder

2 or more cloves of garlic, mashed

5 Tbsp. parsley, chopped

½ cup chopped red onion

1. Soak sunflower seeds overnight, and let them sprout for 4 hours the next day.

2. Place them in a food processor with other ingredients.

3. Blend well until smooth. Add water or rejuvelac to desired consistency.

## Raw Applesauce

Raw applesauce, for those who can tolerate fruit, will help restore natural bowel movements to an intestinal system that has been blasted by antibiotics.

1. Cut 1 or 2 apples in quarters, seeds removed.

2. Blend in food processor until smooth. Add a little water or rejuvelac to help blend the apples.

Suggestions for optional additions:

Fresh cranberries in season

Lemon or lime juice and zest, or ½ chopped lemon

Omega-3 fish oil (lemon will disguise the taste)

Powdered herbs or tinctures

1 Tbsp. organic spirulina or chlorella

Ginger powder and/or cinnamon powder to taste

Tiny bit of pomegranate or other juice

Almond meal

Ground flax meal

## Nori rolls or Romaine olls

Spread sheets of nori seaweed with all sorts of things: roll ingredients together like sushi and eat like a hot dog. Use romaine leaves in similar fashion. Ideas for tasty rolls are:

- Guacamole covered with alfalfa sprouts and shredded, slivered, or julienned carrots and/or cucumbers and chopped tomatoes

- Green salads with sugar-free salad dressing and pâté

- Sunflower pâté, slivered or shredded carrots, red peppers, and/or cucumbers, chopped greens, and slivered olives

Add a few sugar pod peas to rolls if desired.

## Spring Dandelion Salad

Pick a quantity of small dandelion leaves.

Rinse greens.

Toss with minced garlic and olive oil.

Delicious!

## Generic Salad Dressing

The possible combinations for salad dressings are endless. It only takes minutes to concoct a tasty salad dressing. Experiment with proportions to taste. If you come up with a good combination, write it down.

Blend together:

* Olive oil

* Lemon or lime juice

* Water or rejuvelac as consistency dictates

* Fresh or dried green herbs such as basil, parsley, oregano, cilantro, dill, chives, marjoram, mint, sage, or thyme

* A little garlic

* Nuts or seeds: left-over almond, sesame, or sunflower seed mush, raw tahini, sprouted sunflower seeds, pâté, other nuts or sprouted legumes

* Sweetener (optional): soaked raisins, or dates

* Seaweed such as kelp, dulse or nori powder or flakes

* Strong spices such as ginger, mustard, paprika, cayenne

## Beets

Though beets are better juiced or raw, other methods of preparation may provide more variety, especially if you are doing a "beet cure." For a beet cure you could use up to 5 pounds of beets for one day. Suggestions for beets:

- Grate raw, peeled beets for salad. Sprinkle with lemon juice.

- Steam whole beets until tender (for about 25-30 minutes). Large beets may need to be cut in half. Run cooked beets under cold water to see if skins slide off. If skin does not come off easily, return the beets to the steamer until they are done. When they are cooked, remove the skins, root, and stem ends. Cooked beets will keep in the refrigerator overnight.

Serving Suggestions:

- Cut cooked beets into slices or small cubes and season with fresh lemon juice.

- Mash the cooked beets with a little ground cardamom and lemon juice.


## Simple Cold Borscht (Cooked Beets)

8 medium sized beets, peeled, halved, and sliced thinly

7 cups water

Juice of 3 fresh lemons, strained to remove seeds

3 garlic cloves

3/4 cup plain low-fat yogurt (optional)

1 small cucumber, peeled and cut into thin slices

Minced fresh dill or chives

1. Add beets to water, bring to a boil, and simmer for 30 min-

utes.

2. Add the lemon juice and simmer, uncovered, for another 20 minutes.

3. Remove from heat and add garlic.

4. When mixture has cooled, remove the garlic.

5. Place 2 Tbsp. yogurt, if desired, into the center of each soup bowl and add soup.

6. Top with sliced cucumber and minced dill or chives.

## Immunity Soup

(Note: astragalus pieces, fresh burdock pieces and seaweed are good to have on hand to add to other soups)

8 cups filtered water

3 Tbsp. sesame seeds

2 Tbsp. extra virgin coconut oil

One 12-inch piece of burdock root chopped

One 1-1/2 inch piece of ginger grated

1 whole bulb or more of garlic, minced

2 or 3 Tbsp. dry hijiki, dulse or other seaweed

2 cups soaked dried shiitake mushrooms, sliced (keep soak water)

1 large soaked dried reishi mushroom

5 or more pieces of dried astragalus root

1 cup or more chopped green leafy vegetables (spinach, nettles, collards, kale, or dandelion greens)

3 Tbsp. white miso

4 green onions, chopped

4 sprigs fresh cilantro, chopped

1. Bring water to a boil.

2. In a skillet, sauté sesame seeds in coconut oil for a few minutes.

3. Add burdock root, ginger, garlic and hijiki and sauté until tender.

4. Add these to the boiling water.

5. Add astragalus, mushrooms, and soaking water, then turn heat to low and let simmer for 15 minutes.

6. Add green vegetables and simmer until cooked.

7. Remove from heat, let mixture cool for a few minutes.

8. Add miso and mix well.

9. Sprinkle each bowl with green onions and cilantro.


## Garlic Super Soup

Try this blast of "Russian penicillin." This recipe makes enough for 4 servings.

25 garlic cloves, unpeeled

3 Tbsp. olive oil

2 onions, chopped

Fresh thyme

25 garlic cloves, peeled

3 cups water or vegetable stock

½ cup plain yogurt

½ cup grated Parmesan cheese (optional)

4 lemon wedges

1. Preheat oven to 350°.

2. Place unpeeled garlic in small container, add olive oil and toss to cover cloves.

3. Bake for 45 minutes.

4. Cool the cloves.

5. Remove skins from garlic cloves.

6. In a large pot, add enough olive oil for cooking onions and thyme.

7. Cook over medium heat until onions are translucent.

8. Add garlic cloves, both the cooked and the raw, and cook for 3 minutes.

9. Add water or stock, cover pot and simmer for about 20 minutes until garlic is soft.

10. Puree entire mix in blender.

11. Add yogurt and reheat.

12. Serve with parmesan and lemon wedge.

I hope I have been able to convey the possibilities of food as a major healing agent. Adoption of a diet containing largely living foods not only heals the body but, perhaps more importantly, energizes the all-powerful mind that ultimately creates and directs all healing. It offers a way to feel better, perhaps even joyful and energized.

# Appendix B

## The Gerson Program: Detoxification and Hyperalimentation

The Gerson program is the gold standard for restorative diets. Though many people find it hard to stick with such a regimen it is, nevertheless, a good reference point for other dietary therapies. People have healed their Lyme disease following this diet (as reported in the Gerson literature).

Gerson considered salt to be a poison in the body because it inhibits the formation of enzymes, whereas potassium activates enzymes. Restoration of the proper ratio of potassium requires restriction of salt and sodium in foods. An enormous quantity of fresh juices combined with potassium supplementation will restore potassium levels and neutralize and force excretion of salt. This super nutrition requires hourly preparation and drinking of organically grown fruit and vegetable juices along with simply cooked vegetables. Of the juices, carrot is the most frequently used. Below are some of the basic principles of the Gerson program.

### Nutritional Supplements Recommended On the Gerson Diet

- Lugol's solution for iodine

- Coenzyme Q10 supplement in lieu of raw liver juice (no longer safe to consume)

- Pancreatic enzyme tablets

- Potassium supplementation
- Thyroid extract
- Niacin for detoxing
- Hydrochloric acid HCl and pepsin for digestion

Additional highly recommended supplements include:

Bee pollen for nutritional stimulation

Royal jelly

B12 injections

Vitamin C

## The Diet

Patients are put on a vegetarian diet which includes, besides juices, oatmeal and orange juice for breakfast and steamed vegetables for other meals. Only organic foods are consumed. Foods fall into three categories: desirable foods, foods for occasional use, and prohibited foods

## Desirable Foods

- Fresh, organically grown fruits and vegetables, including potatoes
- Freshly made, each time, fruit and vegetable juices 13 times per day (8 ounces each time)
- Fruit and vegetable salads
- Special soup (Hippocrates soup)
- Oatmeal
- Fresh garden herbs

A study of the foods eaten most often by 200 cancer patients who experienced spontaneous regressions revealed that over 70% of them ate the following foods, in descending order of frequency:

Broccoli

Leeks

Cauliflower

Onions

Legumes

Carrots

Brussels sprouts

Beet roots

Squash

Apples

Pears

Apricots

Whole grain cereals

Cantaloupe

Grapes

Tomatoes

## Foods to Use Not More than Once or Twice a Month

- Frozen vegetables without added salt, fat or chemicals

- Bread containing up to 20% whole rye or whole wheat flour, refined as little as possible

- Buckwheat or potato pancakes as long as they contain no baking powder or baking soda

- Unadulterated nonfat milk, nonfat herbal teas

After a person has been on the diet for a while some allowance is made for personal choice of meat, fish, eggs, nuts, etc.

- Popcorn without salt or fat

- Brown or wild rice

- Yams and sweet potatoes

- Maple syrup, raw brown sugar, unsulfured black strap molasses, not to exceed two tsps./day

## Forbidden Foods

- All processed, canned, or manufactured foods

- Refined carbohydrates such as refined white and brown sugars, wheat flour and pasta

- Pineapples and berries if allergic reactions occur

- All oils and fats except fresh raw organic flax seed

- Rich foods such as nuts, seeds, and avocados

- Cucumbers because they do not combine well with the juices

- Dairy products such as cheese

- Irritating spices such as the various peppers and paprika, basil and oregano

- Legumes, including all soy products, soybeans, and other dried legumes

- Sprouted beans and seeds, including alfalfa because they suppress the immune system and can lead to arthritic symptoms

- Mushrooms

- Mustard and carrot greens

## Other Stipulations

- No smoking, alcohol or caffeine, including coffee and tea substitutes

- No fluoride products

- Coffee enemas twice a day to stimulate intestinal function and liver enzymes for detoxification

- Thyroid extracts to strengthen thyroid function

- Limited water drinking, as it dilutes stomach acid

## Cooking of Vegetables

Since enzymes die at 140°, vegetables should be cooked very slowly in their own juice or in a minimum of water or soup stock over low heat for up to an hour or two in a pan with a tight fitting lid (no pressure cookers). Since onions, leeks, or tomatoes stay moist while cooking, they may be added to provide cooking liquid. Beets and potatoes are cooked in their jackets, scrubbed but not peeled or scraped. The steamed vegetables will keep overnight in refrigerator.

## Hippocrates Special Soup

This special soup is a staple of the Gerson diet, eaten at both lunch and dinner. The vegetables are cooked slowly, as above, and then put in a food grinder to make a thick, creamy soup. This recipe makes enough to last up to two days.

One medium celery root or three or four stalks of celery

A small amount of parsley

1-1/2 pounds or more of tomatoes

Two medium onions

One medium parsley root if available

Two small leeks or extra medium sized onions

Several cloves of garlic

1 pound potatoes

## Gerson Recipes for Other Foods

The Gerson program also allows for various juices, salads and fresh salad dressings, cooked vegetable dishes, potato recipes, vegetarian loaves, dairy dishes when suitable, breads made with organic rye and only a very little whole wheat, and occasional desserts made of fruits, raw or stewed.

## Juicers

Gerson recommends the Norwalk juicer, a triturator grinder/press combination juicer. The K & K juicer is also recommended, although one would have to look for a used one since no one is making them anymore. The second best juicers are masticating juicers which chew up the vegetables and extract juices in one step. Examples of this are the Champion juicer and the Green Star. The Green Star is preferable to the Champion because it does a much better job with greens.

The common cheap, centrifugal juicers are not suitable for a serious healing program: Gerson patients who used these juicers were not as successful in their therapy.

## Conditions Not Totally Helped By This Diet

While this diet can produce miraculous effects for a wide range of illnesses, particularly the illnesses of modern civilization such as cancer, heart disease, and diabetes, some conditions do not respond so readily to it. The Gerson Institute reports limited success with:

Brain cancer

Bone metastases

Open breast cancer lesions

Acute childhood leukemias (age-onset leukemias do respond well)

Multiple myeloma

Long-term prednisone treatment and/or chemotherapy

## "Not Curable" With the Gerson Method:

- Amyotrophic lateral sclerosis (ALS): they achieved some success when they were able to obtain liver juice from healthy young calves. Liver juice is no longer considered safe to use due to widespread use of agricultural chemicals.

- Parkinson's disease.

- Alzheimer's disease if the brain cells are gone or dead: damaged brain cells can be improved or restored.

- Advanced chronic kidney disease: if 20% kidney function remains, the patient can survive if he stays on the diet for life.

- Emphysema: sick tissue can be restored but dead tissue is gone for good.

- Muscular dystrophy no longer responds to the treatment.

## The Mental Aspect of the Program

A final aspect of the Gerson program is the mental part: Persons following the diet also work to eliminate negative psychological states of mind in various ways:

- Relaxation techniques

- Visualizations for self-healing

- Simple meditations
- Constant use of affirmations
- Developing the creative power of the right brain
- Overcoming negative family issues
- Positive actions in all situations
- Full understanding of the Gerson program
- Removing pain with use of coffee enemas and detoxification
- Reinforcement through relief of symptoms

# Resources/Links

## Home Ozone Setup

### Oxygen Tanks

Tanks purchased from a welding supply store are considerably cheaper than medical oxygen tanks. The oxygen in the tank is exactly the same as that in medical tanks. It is important that any tank be free of oil, as that could be hazardous. You need at least a 20 lb. tank (or larger if you do regular ozone saunas). Tank refills are inexpensive.

### Medical Ozone Generator

Ozone generators are available at **www.promolife.com.**

More expensive units are available from **www.ozoneservices. com.** These units usually come with a regulator and a small medical oxygen tank (quite inadequate for frequent use), as well as a lot of useful attachments.

Inexpensive Chinese units are available on EBay. If you purchase one of these, be sure that the oxygen source is from a tank of pure oxygen rather than ambient air, and that the unit has no built-in air pump (not needed or desired). They are advertised for the tropical fish industry, a very fragile population. People have reported these machines to be accurate for home use. The only problem with some of them is that they put out a high-pitched whine while in use. There is probably an easy solution to this. These machines do not come with tubing or regulator.

## Fiberglass Sauna Tent

The tent material must be of fiberglass to withstand ozone. If you can't find one of these, a regular steam sauna tent will do, but it will be subject to deterioration over time. Distilled water for the sauna is heated in a modified Japanese rice cooker. I have found that most of these do not last very long because they are cheaply made. The best cooker I have found came from **http://www.ib-3health.com/**.

## Pediatric Regulator

If your machine does not come with a pediatric regulator, you will need to purchase one. The regulator fits onto the oxygen tank to regulate the flow of oxygen into the ozone machine. A regulator with brass innards is fairly inexpensive. Anything besides brass will eventually deteriorate from the ozone.

**http://www.cramerdeckermedical.com/product. php?product_id=583**. You need the "barb only" model.

CGA 540 Regulator 0-4, barb only, calibrations beginning at 1/32 LPM

MSRP prices starting about $40

Part Number: AREG540x

## Tubing

Tubing from the oxygen tank to ozone machine can be similar to that used in food and beverage dispensing equipment. These items are available from **www.usplastic.com**.

Tygon® Beverage Tubing 1/4" inner dimension; 3/8" outer dimension; 1/16" wall

Working pressure - 36 PSI @ 73° F

Item #: 57220  Price: $1.09 per foot

Tubing from the ozone machine itself must be silicone low temperature tubing to withstand the ozone:

Silicon® Tubing: 1/4" inner dimension x 3/8" outer dimension

Working pressure - 5 @ 70° F

Item #: 54033   Price: $0.73 per foot

Manufacturer: Newage

## Connectors for Tubing:

Quick Disconnects:

3/8" to 1/4" Polyethylene Quick Disconnect 2 5/8" Overall length

3/4" connection length

Item #: 64026   Price: $1.94

Made of polyethylene; fits snugly; comes apart easily. Useful tool in flexible tubing systems

Manufacturer: Bel-Art Products

## Catheters

Catheters for rectal or vaginal insufflations may be purchased from a medical supply store. The so-called French catheters up to 14" work well.

## Far-Infrared Sauna

Therassage is a low EMF (electromagnetic frequency) portable sauna: **www.therassage.com**. Avoid saunas that do not mention EMF qualities.

## Masks for Exercise with Oxygen

http://www.deltaoxygensystems.com/catalog/i101.html
http://www.deltaoxygensystems.com/id99.html

## Binaural Beat CDs and Software

Monroe Institute: http://www.monroeinstitute.org/resources/hemi-sync

Binaural beat downloads: http://www.monroeinstitute.org/catalog/audio-downloads

Mind Stereo software for creating binaural beats:

http://www.transparentcorp.com/products/mindstereo/index.php

## Himalayan Institute *Pranayama* on YouTube

*Ujjayi* https://yogainternational.com/article/view/ujjayi-pranayama-victory-breath

http://youtu.be/iy4PRzHP9XM

*Bhastrika* http://youtu.be/J4nf-NISmJw

*Kapalabhati* http://youtu.be/B6bnFlVkKrE

## Reasonably Priced Organic Essential Oils

Mountain Rose Herbs: http://www.mountainroseherbs.com/catalog

Ancient Ways Botanicals: http://ancientwaysbotanicals.com/

New Directions Aromatics: http://www.newdirectionsaromatics.com/

Aroma Tools for tools to use with essential oils: **www.aro-matools.com**

Low-Dose Naltrexone Information: **http://www.low-dosenaltrexone.org/#additional_info**

## Stephen Buhner

**http://planetthrive.com/**

Website for his *Healing Lyme* book: **http://buhnerhealin-glyme.com/about/**

## Dr. Klinghardt

**http://www.klinghardtacademy.com/Lyme-Disease/**

Dr. Mercola's 7 part interview with Dr. Klinghardt begins here: **http://www.youtube.com/watch?v=QRatMUJifaQ \**

## Dr. Mercola

Searchable website full of useful research and current information on numerous topics: **http://mercola.com/**

## Visualizations

Many people use scripts from Belleruth Naparstek: **http://belleruthnaparstek.com/**

## Product Resources

Azure Standard for bulk and natural foods: **http://www.azurestandard.com/**

## Movies about Food

*The Gerson Miracle* documentary: **http://www.youtube. com/watch?v=sbIixJI_oa4&wide=1**

*Forks over Knives*

*Fat, Sick and Nearly Dead*

*Food Matters*

*Vegucated*

*Hungry for Change*

*The Beautiful Truth: The World's Simplest Cure for Cancer*

*Dying to Have Known: The Evidence behind Natural Healing*

## Other Information Sources/Websites

• Excellent article about Lyme in the New Yorker magazine, July 1, 2013: **http://www.newyorker.com/ reporting/2013/07/01/130701fa_fact_specter?printable =true&currentPage=all**

• Amy Yasko: *Autism: Pathways to Recovery*. Bethel, ME: Neurological Research Institute, 2009. This excellent book is available for free download at **http://www.holisticheal. com/media/downloads/autism-pathways-to-recovery- book.pdf**

• D. S. Myhill on chronic fatigue: **http://www.ei-resource. org/articles/chronic-fatigue-syndrome-articles/the- methylation-cycle/.**

• Rich van Konynenburg. "Suggestions for Treatment of Chronic Fatigue Syndrome (CFS) based on the Glutathione Depletion—Methylation Cycle Block Hypothesis for the Pathogenesis of CFS: The Simple Approach." **http://about- mecfs.org/Trt/TrtGSHMethISimple.aspx.**

- Majid Ali. "Seven Aspects of Oxygen and Oxidation." **http: http://www.majidali.com/seven.htm** .

- Mary Enig. "Coconut: in Support of Good Health in the 21st Century." **http://www.snc.sg/about-us/ publications/coconut-oil/coconut-in-support-of-good-health-in-the-21st-century.**

- Information about medical marijuana: **http://medicalmarijuanadoctors.org/granny-storm-crows-list**

- Dr. William Courtney on medical marijuana: **http://www. youtube.com/watch?v=eRLVyGfGcZs&feature=youtu. be&t=8m11s**

# Bibliography

Ali, Majid. *The Canary and Chronic Fatigue*. 2nd. New York: Life Span Books, 1994.

Altman, Nathaniel. *Oxygen Healing Therapies: For Optimum Health and Vitality*. Rochester, VT: Healing Arts Press, 1998.

—. *The Oxygen Prescription: The Miracle of Oxydative Therapies*. Rochester, VT: Healing Arts Press, 2007.

Appleton, Nancy. *Lick the Sugar Habit*. 2nd. New York: Avery, 1988.

—. *Suicide by Sugar*. Garden City Park, NY: Square One Publishers, 2009.

Bailey, Steven, and Larry Jr Trivieri. *Juice Alive: The Ultimate Guide to Juicing Remedies*. Garden City Park, NY: Square One Publishers, 2006.

Ballantyne, Sarah. *The Paleo Approach: Reverse Autoimmune Disease and Heal Your Body*. Las Vegas, NV: Victory Belt Publishing, 2014.

Barnes, Broda. *Hypothyroidism: The Unsuspected Illness*. New York: Harper Collins, 1976.

Berendt, Joachim-Ernst. *The World of Sound Nada Brahma: Music and the Landscape of Consciousness*. Translated by Helmut Bredigkeit. Rochester, VT: Destiny Books, 1991.

Berkson, D. Lindsey. *Healthy Digestion the Natural Way: Preventing and Healing Heartburn, Constipation, Gas, Diarrhea, Inflammatory Bowel and Gallbladder Diseases, Ulcers, Irritable Bowel Syndrome, and More*. New York: Wiley, 2000.

Bernstein, *Richard K. Dr. Bernstein's Diabetes Solution: The Complete Guide to Achieving Normal Blood Sugars*. 4th Updated. New

York: Little, Brown and Company, 2011.

Biser, Sam. *A Layman's Guide to Curing with Cayenne and its Herbal Partners*. Van Nuys, CA: Save Your Life Videos, Inc., 1999.

Black, Jessica. *The Anti-Inflammation Diet and Recipe Book: Protect Yourself and Your Family from Heart Disease, Arthritis, Diabetes, Allergies - and More*. Alameda, CA: Hunter House, 2006.

Bocci, Velio. **Ozone: A New Medical Drug**. New York: Springer, 2005.

Boyle, Wade, and Andre Saine. *Lectures in Naturopathic Hydrotherapy*. Sandy, OR: Eclectic Medical Publications, 1988.

Braun, Linda. *Spirulina: Food for the Future*. Beltsville, MD: US Dept. of Agriculture, Aquaculture Information Center, 1988.

Brown, Richard, and Patricia Gerbarg. *The Healing Power of the Breath: Simple Techniques to Reduce Stress and Anxiety, Enhance Concentration, and Balance Your Emotions*. Boston: Shambhala, 2012.

Buhner, Stephen Harrod. *Healing Lyme: Natural Healing and Prevention of Lyme Borreliosis and its Coinfections*. Randolph, VT: Raven Press, 2005.

—. *Herbal Antibiotics*. Storey Publishing, LLC, 1999.

—. *Herbs for Hepatitis C and the Liver*. Pownal, VT: Storey Books, 2000.

Calabro, Rose Lee. *Living in the Raw*. Santa Cruz: Rose Publishing, 1998.

Calbom, Cherie, and Maureen Keane. *Juicing for Life: A Guide to the Health Benefits of Fresh Fruit and Vegetable Juicing*. Garden City Park, NY: Avery Publishing Group, 1992.

Campbell-McBride, Natasha. *Gut and Psychology Syndrome: Natural Treatment for Autism, Dyspraxia, A.D.D., Dyslexia, A.D.H.D., Depression, Schizophrenia*. Revised & enlarged edition . Cambridge: Medinform Publishing, 2010.

Challem, Jack Joseph. *Spirulina: What it is, and the Health Benefits it Can Give You*. New York: McGraw Hill, 1999.

Christopher, John. *School of Natural Healing*. Orem, Utah: Christopher Publications., n.d.

Cohen, Kenneth. *The Way of Qi Gong: The Art and Science of Chinese Energy Healing*. New York: Ballentine Books, 1997.

Cott, Allan. *Fasting: The Ultimate Diet*. Winter Park, FLA: Hastings House, 1997.

Courdain, Loren. *The Paleo Diet Revised: Lose Weight and Get Healthy by Eating the Foods You Were Designed to Eat*. Revised Edition. New York: Houghton Mifflin Harcourt, 2010.

Cousins, Norman. *Anatomy of an Illness as Perceived by the Patient: Reflections on Healing and Regeneration*. Boston:: Shambhala Publications, 1991.

—. Head First: *The Biology of Hope and the Healing Power of the Human Spirit*. New York: Penguin Books, 1989.

Crocker, Pat. *The Juicing Bible*. 2nd. Toronto: Robert Rose, 2008.

Crook, W. J. *The Yeast Connection: A Medical Breakthrough*. Updated revised. New York: Vintage Books, 1986.

de Baïracli Levy, Juliette. *Common Herbs for Natural Health*. New York: Schocken Books, 1974.

Dean, Carolyn, MD. *Death by Modern Medicine*. Belleville, ONT: Matrix Verite, 2005.

Demos, John N. *Getting Started with Neurofeedback*. New York: W. W. Norton, 2005.

Douglas, William Campbell. *Hydrogen Peroxide: Medical Miracle*. Atlanta: Second Opinion Publishing, 1992.

Duke, James A. *Dr. Duke's Essential Herbs: 13 Vital Herbs You Need to Disease-Proof Your Body, Boost Your Energy, Lengthen Your Life*. Emmaus, PA: Rodale Books, 1999.

—. *Handbook of Medicinal Herbs*. Boca Raton, FL: CRC, 2002.

—. *The Green Pharmacy Guide to Healing Foods: Proven Natural*

*Remedies to Treat and Prevent More Than 80 Common Health Concerns*. Emmaus, PA: Rodale, 2009.

—. *The Green Pharmacy Herbal Handbook: Your Comprehensive Reference to the Best Herbs for Healing*. Emmaus, PA: Rodale/Reach, 2000.

Elias, Thomas S., and Peter A. Dykeman. *Edible Wild Plants: A North American Field Guide*. Sterling Publishing Co. Inc., 1990.

Enig, Mary. Know Your Fats: *The Complete Primer for Understanding the Nutrition of Fats, Oils and Cholesterol*. Silver Spring, MD: Bethesda Press, 2000.

Erasmus, Udo. *Fats and Oils*. Vancouver, BC: Alive Books, 1989.

Fried, Robert. *Breathe Well, Be Well: A Program to Relieve Stress, Anxiety, Asthma, Hypertension, Migraine, and Other Disorders for Better Health*. New York: Wiley, 1999.

Fuhrman, Joel. *Eat to Live: The Amazing Nutrient-Rich Program for Fast and Sustained Weight Loss*. Revised Edition. New York: Little, Brown and Company, 2011.

Gerard, Robert V. **DNA Healing Techniques: Tools for Physical and Emotional Self-Healing**. 3rd. Coarsegold, CA: Oughten Foundation, Inc., 1999.

Gerson, Charlotte, and Morton Walker. *The Gerson Therapy: the Amazing Nutritional Program for Cancer and Other Illnesses*. Stamford, CT: Freelance Communications, 2001.

Gerson, Max. *A Cancer Therapy: Results of Fifty Cases and the Cure of Advanced Cancer by Diet Therapy*. 6th. Gerson Institute, 1958.

Goulart, F. S. *"Are You Sugar Smart?" American Fitness*, April 1991: 34-38.

Grieves, Maud. *A Modern Herbal: The Medicinal, Culinary, Cosmetic and Economic Properties, Cultivation and Folk-Lore of Herbs, Grasses, Fungi, Shrubs & Trees with Their Modern Scientific Uses*. 2 vols. New York: Dover, 1971.

Hobbs, Christopher. *Natural Therapy for Your Liver: Herbs and Other Natural Remedies for a Healthy Liver*. Revised and updated.

New York, CA: Avery, 2002.

Howell, Edward. *Enzyme Nutrition*. Wayne, NJ: Avery Publishing Group, 1985.

Jensen, Bernard. *Empty Harvest: Understanding the Link Between our Food, our Immunity, and our Planet*. Garden City: Avery, 1995.

—. *Healing Power of Chlorophyll from Plant Life: Magic Survival Kit Book*. 2nd. Jensen Enterprises, 1973.

Kallas, John. *Edible Wild Plants: Wild Foods From Dirt To Plate (The Wild Food Adventure Series, Book 1)*. Layton, UT: Gibbs Smith, 2010.

Kavanaugh, Nicole,. "Selected Antimicrobial Essential Oils Eradicate Pseudomonas spp. and Staphylococcus aureus Biofilms." *Appl Environ Microbiol* 78, no. 11 (June 2012): 4057-4061.

Kirschner, H. E. *Nature's Healing Grasses*. Riverside: H. C. White Publications, 1960.

Kirschner, H. E., MD. *Live Food Juices for Vim, Vigor, Vitality, Long Life*. Monrovia, CA: H. E. Kirschner Publiucations, 1977.

Konlee, Mark. *How to Reverse Immune Dysfunction*. West Allis, WI: Keep Hope Alive, 1996.

—. *Immune Restoration Handbook*. West Allis, WI: Keep Hope Alive, 2003.

*The Gerson Miracle*. DVD. Directed by Stephen Kroschel. Produced by Haines, SK: Kroschel Films. 2004.

Kulvinskas, Viktoras. *Sprout for the Love of Everybody*. Wethersfield, CT: Omango D' Press, 1988.

Kurt, Schnaubelt<. *Medical Aromatherapy: Healing with Essential Oils*. Berkeley, CA: Frog Books/North Atlantic, 1999.

Larson, Joan Mathews. *Depression Free Naturally: 7 Weeks to Eliminating Anxiety, Despair, Fatigue, and Anger from Your Life*. New York: Ballentine Books, 1999.

Larson, Stephen. *The Healing Power of Neurofeedback: The Revolutionary LENS Technique for Restoring Optimal Brain Function.* Rochester, VT: Healing Arts Press, 2006.

Levine, Barbara Hoberman. *Your Body Believes Every Word You Say: The Language of the Body/Mind Connection.* 2nd. Boulder Creek, CA: Aslan Publishing, 1991.

*Low Dose Naltrexone.* n.d. http://www.lowdosenaltrexone.org/ (accessed May 2011).

Marz, Russell B. *Medical Nutrition from Marz.* 2nd. Portland, OR: Quiet Lion Press, 1999.

Mate, Gabor. *When the Body Says No: Exploring the Stress-Disease Connection.* New York: Wiley, 2011.

Mateljan, George. *The World's Healthiest Foods, Essential Guide for the Healthiest Way of Eating.* New York: GMF Publishing, 2006.

Maurice, Messegue. *Health Secrets of Plants and Herbs.* London: Pan Books, Ltd., 1983.

McCabe, Ed. *Flood Your Body with Oxygen: Therapy for our Polluted World.* Miami Shores: Energy Publications, 2003.

—. *Oxygen Therapies: A New Way of Approaching Disease.* Miami Shores: Energy Publications, 1988.

McClelland, Jennifer. *The Right Blend: Blender-only Raw Food Recipes.* Fruitland, ID: Be Deliciously Healthy, 2003.

McConnaughey, Evelyn. *Sea Vegetables: Harvesting Guide and Cookbook.* Happy Camp, CA: Naturgraph Publishers, Inc., 1985.

Meyerowitz, Steve. *Power Juices, Super Drinks: Quick, Delicious Recipes to Prevent and Reverse Disease.* New York: Kensington Publishing, 2000.

—. *Wheatgrass Nature's Finest Medicine: The Complete Guide to Using Grasses to Revitalize Your Health.* 6th. Great Barrington: Sproutman Publications, 1999.

Moritz, Andreas. *The Liver and Gallbladder Miracle Cleanse: An*

*All-Natural, At-Home Flush to Purify and Rejuvenate Your Body.* Berkeley, CA: Ulysses Press, 2007.

Mowrey, Daniel B. Mowrey. *Next Generation Herbal Medicine.* 2 Rev Sub edition . Keats Publishing, 1991.

MT/CFS Methylation Forum. *Food Nutritional Data.* n.d. http://me-cfsmethylation.com/viewtopic.php?f=4&t=38 (accessed December 3, 2010).

Naparstek, Belleruth. *Staying Well With Guided Imagery: How to Harness the Power of Your Imagination for Health and Healing.* New York: Warner Books, 1994.

Nyerges, Christopher. *Guide to Wild Foods and Useful Plants.* Chicago: Chicago Review Press, 1999.

Olson, S. A. *The Jade Emperor's Mind Seal Classic: The Taoist Guide to Health, Longevity, and Immortality.* Rochester, VT: Inner Traditions, 2003.

Perque. "How to do an Ascorbate (Vitamin C) Calibration Protocol ("C Flush") to Determine Individual, Functional Need for Ascorbate." http://www.perque.com/uploads/Pt_Ascorbate_Slush_FIN.pdf, n.d.

Pert, Candace. *Molecules of Emotion: Why you Feel the Way you Feel.* New York: Simon and Schuster, 1997.

Pizzorno, Joseph E., and Michael T. Murray. *Textbook of Natural Medicine.* 2nd. New York: Harcourt Health Sciences Group, 1999.

Pressman, Saul. *The Story of Ozone.* Langley, BC: http://www.o3center.org/Articles/TheStoryofOzone.html, n.d.

Quillin, Patrick. *Beating Cancer with Nutrition.* 4th. Carlsbad, CA: Nutrition Times Press, 2001.

Reid, D. *The Complete Book of Chinese Health & Healing: Guarding the Three Treasures.* Boston: Shambhala, 1994.

Ross, Julia. *The Diet Cure: The 8-Step Program to Rebalance Your Body Chemistry and End Food Cravings, Weight Problems, and Mood Swings—Now.* New York: Penguin, 2000.

Saraswati, Srimat Swami Shivananda. *Yogic Therapy or Yogic Way to Cure Diseases*. Assam: Brahmachari Yogeshwar, Umachal Yogashram, Kamakhya, Gauhati-10, 1978.

Schnaubelt, Kurt. *Advanced Aromatherapy: The Science of Essential Oil Therapy*. 1st Ameericsn. Rochester, VT: Healing Arts Press, 1998.

—. *The Healing Intelligence of Essential Oils: The Science of Advanced Aromatherapy*. Rochester, VT: Healing Arts Press, 2011.

Shealy, Norman. "The Reality of EEG and Neurochemical Responses to Photostimulation Part 1." *In Light Years Ahead*, edited by Brian Breiling, 165-84. Berkeley: Celestial Arts, 1996.

Siebert, Al, Ph.D. *The Survivor Personality: Why Some People are Stronger, Smarter, and More Skillful at Handling Life's Difficulties . . . and How You Can Be Too*. New York: Perigee/Berkley Publishing Group, 1996.

Sigal, Lance. *The Earthrise Spirulina Cookbook: Make Great Meals with a Superfood*. Bloomington, IN: Authorhouse, 2005.

Simonton, O. Carl, M.D., Reid Henson, and Brenda Hampton. *The Healing Journey*. New York. New York: Bantam, 1994.

Sojourner, Caroline. *Total Healing to the Limits of Living: Awakening and Engaging the Healing Energies of the Tree of Life*. Lake Oswego, OR: Black Wolf Matrix, 2009.

Soria, Cherie. *Angel Foods: Healthy Recipes for Heavenly Bodies*. Heartstar Productions, 1996.

—. *Angel Foods: Healthy Recipes for Heavenly Bodies*. Revised. Summertown, TN: Book Publishing Company, 2003.

—. *Raw Food For Dummies*. New York: For Dummies/Wiley, 2012.

Stone, Randolph. *Health-Building: The Conscious Art of Living Well*. TN: Book Publishing Company, 1999.

Storl, Wolf D. *Healing Lyme Disease Naturally: History, Analysis, and Treatments*. Berkeley: North Atlantic Books, 2010.

Suzuki, T. et al, eds. *Aces in Mercury Toxicology*. New York: Plenum Press, 1991.

Sylver, Nenah. *The Holistic Handbook of Sauna Therapy*. New York: Center for Frequency Education, 2003.

Thayer, Samuel. *Edible Wild Plants: Wild Foods From Dirt To Plate (The Wild Food Adventure Series, Book 1)*. Birchwood, WI: Forager's Harvest Press, 2006.

Thrash, Agatha, and Calvin Thrash. *Home Remedies: Hydrotherapy, Massage, Charcoal and Other Simple Remedies*. Seale, AL: Thrash Publications, 1981.

Transparent Corporation. "*The Science behind Mind Stereo.*" Transparent Corp. n.d. http://www.transparentcorp.com/products/mindstereo/science.php (accessed October 18, 2008).

USDA Agricultural Research Service. *Nutritive Value of Foods, Home and Garden Bulletin No. 72* (HG-72). n.d. http://www.ars.usda.gov/Services/docs.htm?docid=6282 (accessed December 3, 2010).

Vanderhaeghe, L. R. and P. J. D. Bouic. *The Immune System Cure: Optimize Your Immune system in 30 Days--The Natural Way!* New York: Kensington Books, 1999.

von Ardenne, Manfred. *Oxygen Multistep Therapy: Physiological and Technical Foundations*. New York: Thieme New York, 1987.

Walker, Norman. *Raw Vegetable Juices*. New York: Jove Publications, 1970.

Ware, James R., trans. *Alchemy, Medicine and Religion in the China of A.D. 320: The Nei Pien of Ko Hung*. New York: Dover, 1966.

Weintraub, Skye. *The Parasite Menace: A Complete Guide to the Prevention, Treatment and Elimination of Parasitic Infection*. Woodland Publishing, 2000.

Wigmore, Ann. *The Sprouting Book*. Wayne, NJ: Avery Publishing Group, Inc., 1986.

Wilson, L. D. *Sauna Therapy for Detoxification and Healing*. Prescott,

AZ: LD Wilson Consultants, Inc., 2004.

Winston, David, and Steven Maimes. *Adaptogens: Herbs for Strength, Stamina, and Stress Relief.* Rochester, VT: Healing Arts Press, 2007.

Yasko, Amy. Autism: *Pathways to Recovery.* Bethel, ME: Neurological Research Institute, 2009.

Yogananda, Paramahansa. *Scientific Healing Affirmations.* Los Angeles: Self Realization Fellowship, 1974.

Young, Gary. *Essential Oils Pocket Reference.* Fifth edition. Life Science Publishing, 2011.

# Notes

1   Storl, 2010, 117.

2   Myhill, S. http://www.ei-resource.org/articles/chronic-fatigue-syndrome-articles/the-methylation-cycle/ .

3   Kidd, Paris. "Th1/Th2 Balance: The Hypothesis, Its Limitations, and Implications for Health and Disease." *Alternative Medicine Review,* August 2003.

4   http://articles.mercola.com/sites/articles/archive/2012/09/05/microbes-manipulate-your-mind.aspx?e_cid=20120905_DNL_artNew_1

5   http://articles.mercola.com/sites/articles/archive/2012/05/12/dr-campbell-mcbride-on-gaps.aspx?e_cid=20120520_SNL_MV_1

6   Horner, Christine. "How to Starve Cancer Out of Your Body - Avoid These Top 4 Cancer-Feeding Foods." Jan 14, 2012. http://articles.mercola.com/sites/articles/archive/2012/01/14/dr-christine-horner-interview.aspx (accessed July 1, 2012). http://articles.mercola.com/sites/articles/archive/2012/01/14/dr-christine-horner-interview.aspx

7   http://articles.mercola.com/sites/articles/archive/2012/01/14/dr-christine-horner-interview.aspx

8   Lieber, Charles S. "S-Adenosyl-L-Methionine: Its Role in the Treatment of Liver Disorders." *The American Journal of Clinical Nutrition* 76 (5) (2002): 11835-75.

9   Konynenburg R., "Is Glutathione Depletion An Important Part Of The Pathogenesis Of Chronic Fatigue Syndrome?" Seventh International AACFS Conference. Madison, WI, 2004. See also his list of suggested supplements: http://www.cfsresearch.org/cfs/richvank/augmenting-glutathione-cfs.htm; For further information see the work of Dr. Amy Yasko at: http://me-cfsmethylation.com/viewtopic.php?f=1&t=56.

10  Konynenburg, van, Rich. "Chronic Fatigue Syndrome and Autism." *Townsend Letter for Doctors and Patients*, no. 279 (2006): 84-86.

11  Herzenberg, L. A. "Glutathione Deficiency is Associated with Impaired Survival in HIV Disease." *Proceedings of the National Academy of Sciences* 94 (1997): 1967–72.

12  Yasko, Amy. *Autism: Pathways to Recovery.* Bethel, ME: Neurological Research Institute, 2009. This excellent book is available for free download at http://www.holisticheal.com/media/downloads/autism-pathways-to-recovery-book.pdf

[13] Myhill D. S. http://www.ei-resource.org/articles/chronic-fatigue-syndrome-articles/the-methylation-cycle/.

[14] See also Konynenburg, Rich van. "Suggestions for Treatment of Chronic Fatigue Syndrome (CFS) based on the Glutathione Depletion—Methylation Cycle Block Hypothesis for the Pathogenesis of CFS: The Simple Approach." http://aboutmecfs.org/Trt/TrtGSH-MethISimple.aspx. January 2007 (accessed November 27, 2010).

[15] Dickinson, D. A. et al. "Curcumin Alters Epre and AP-1 Binding Complexes and Elevates Glutamate-Cysteine Ligase Gene Expression." *FASEB J.* 17, no. 3 (2003): 473-475.

[16] Bounous, G., et al. "The Biological Activity of Undenatured Dietary Whey Proteins: Role of Glutathione." *Clinical and Investigative Medicine. Medecine Clinique et Experimentale* 14 (4) 14 (4) (1991): 296-309.

[17] Garcion, E. N. et al. "New Clues about Vitamin D Functions in the Nervous System." *Trends in Endocrinology and Metabolism* 13 (3) (2002): 100-5.

[18] Johnston, C. J. et al. 'Vitamin C Elevates Red Blood Cell Glutathione in Healthy Adults.' *Am J Clin Nutr* 58:103-5, 1993.

[19] Kavanaugh, N., & Ribbeck, K. (2012, June). "Selected Antimicrobial Essential Oils Eradicate Pseudomonas spp. and Staphylococcus aureus Biofilms." *Appl Environ Microbiol,* 78(11), 4057-4061.

[20] Young, 309

[21] Schnaubelt, 2011, 136-7.

[22] Ibid, 138.

[23] Young, 308.

[24] Klinghardt, Dietrich D. "Lyme disease: A Look beyond Antibiotics" http://www.klinghardtacademy.com/images/stories/Lyme_Disease/Lyme_protocol_Jan06.pdf (accessed 2009).

[25] For a serious kidney formula, see Hulda Clark, *The Cure for all Advanced Cancers.*

[26] Ali, Majid. "Seven Aspects of Oxygen and Oxidation." http://www.majidali.com. n.d. http://www.majidali.com/seven.htm (accessed November 22, 2010).

[27] Worthington, Virginia. "Nutritional Quality of Organic Versus Conventional Fruits, Vegetables, and Grains." *Journal of Alternative and Complementary Medicine,* no. 7 (2001): 161-173.

[28] Bouic, P. J. D. "Immunomodulation in HIV/AIDS: The Tygerberg/Stennenbosch University Experience." *AIDS Bulletin* 6 (1997): 18-20.

[29] *Monograph in Alternative Medicine Review*, April, 2001.

[30] Vanderhaeghe, L. R. and P. J. D. Bouic.

[31] Hammell-Dupont, C. et al. "The Stimulation of Hemoglobin Synthesis by Porphyrins." *Biochemical Medicine* 4 (1970): 55-60.

[32] See Chernomorsky, S., and Segelman, A. "Biological Activities of Chlorophyll Derivatives." *New Jersey Medicine* 85 (1988): 669-73.

[33] Shealy, Norman. "The Reality of EEG and Neurochemical Responses to Photostimulation Part 1." *In Light Years Ahead,* edited by Brian Breiling, 165-84. Berkeley: Celestial Arts, 1996, 165-184.

[34] Kimm, S., et al. "Antimutagenic Activity of Chlorophyll to Direct and Indirect-Acting Mutagens and Its Contents in the Vegetables." *Korean Journal of Biochemistry* 14 (1982): 1-7.

[35] Rafsky, H. et al. "The Treatment of Intestinal Diseases with Solutions of Water-Soluble Chlorophyll." *Review of Gastroenterology* 15 (1948): 549-553. 15 (1948): 559-553.

[36] Offenkrantz, W. "Water-Soluble Chlorophyll in the Treatment of Peptic Ulcers of Long Duration." *Review of Gastroenterology* 17 (1950): 359-367.

[37] Richard Kozlenko DPM, PhD M.P.H. et al. "Latest Scientific Research on Spirulina: Effects on the AIDS Virus," *Cancer and the Immune System.* 1998.

[38] *30th Annual Meeting of the Japanese Society for Immunology*, November 2000.

[39] Embry, Ashton. "Multiple Sclerosis - Best Bet Treatment." http://www.direct-ms.org/bestbet.html (accessed December 3, 2010).

[40] Erasmus, 375.

[41] Enig, Mary. "Coconut: in Support of Good Health in the 21st Century." *Progress*. 36th meeting of APCC, 1999. http://www.snc.sg/about-us/publications/coconut-oil/coconut-in-support-of-good-health-in-the-21st-century (accessed May 2012).

[42] Tantibhedhyangkul, P., et al. "Medium-Chain Triglyceride Feeding in Premature Infants: Effects on Calcium and Magnesium Absorption." *Pediatrics* 61 (1987): 537-545.

[43] Eckel, R. H., et al. "Dietary Substitution of Medium-Chain Triglycerides Improves Insulin-Mediated Glucose Metabolism in NIDDM Subjects." *Diabetes* 1992; 41:641-647. 41 (1992): 641-47.

[44] Zakaria, A. A., et al. "In Vivo Antinociceptive and Anti-Inflammatory Activities of Dried and Fermented Processed Virgin Coconut Oil." *Med Princ Pract* 20 (2011): 231-236.

[45] Monserrat, A.J., et al. "Protective Effect of Coconut Oil on Renal Necrosis Occurring in Rats Fed a Methyl-Deficient Diet." *Ren Fail* 17 (1995): 525-37; Mizushima, T., et al. "Pre-

vention of Hyperlipidemic Acute Pancreatitis During Pregnancy With Medium-Chain Triglyceride [18] Nutritional Support." *Int J Pancreatol* 23 (1998): 187-92; Kono, H., et al. "Medium-Chain Triglycerides Enhance Secretory Iga Expression in Rat Intestine after Administration of Endotoxin." *Am J Physiol Gastrointest Liver Physiol* 286 (2004): G1081-G1089.

[46] http://www.jeannerose.net/articles/lyme_disease.html

[47] Fahey, Jed et al. "Broccoli Sprouts: An Exceptionally Rich Source of Inducers of Enzymes That Protect Against Chemical Carcinogens." *Proc. Natl. Acad. Sci. USA* 94 (September 1997): 10367-72.

[48] Jones, D. P. et al. "Glutathione in Foods listed in the National Cancer Institute's Health Habits and History Food Frequency Questionnaire." *Nutr Cancer* 17: 57-75, 1992.

[49] Wigmore, 1986, 109.

[50] Duke, James. *Handbook of Medicinal Herbs*. Boca Raton, FL: CRC, 2002.

[51] Ibid.

[52] Ibid.

[53] Berga, S. L., et al. "Endocrine and Chronobiological Effects of Fasting in Women." *Fertil Steril.* 2001 May; 75(5):926-32; Brehm, B. J., et al. "A Randomized Trial Comparing a Very Low Carbohydrate Diet and a Calorie-Restricted Low Fat Diet on Body Weight and Cardiovascular Risk Factors in Healthy Women." *J Clin Endocrinol Metab.* 2003 Apr;88(4):1617-23; Faintuch, J., et al. "Changes in Body Fluid and Energy Compartments During Prolonged Hunger Strike." *J. Nutrition* 2001 Feb; 17 (2):100-4; Seim, H. C., et al. "Electrocardiographic Findings Associated With Very Low Calorie Dieting." *Int J Obes Relat Metab Disord* 1995 Nov; 19(11):817-9.

[54] Seim, H. C. et al. *Int J Obes Relat Metab Disord* 1995 Nov; 19(11):817-9; "Electrocardiographic Findings Associated With Very Low Calorie Dieting."

[55] http://articles.mercola.com/sites/articles/archive/2013/02/11/all-fruit-diet.aspx?e_cid=20130211_DNL_art_1&utm_source=dnl&utm_medium=email&utm_campaign=20130211

[56] Kidd, Paris. "Th1/Th2 Balance: The Hypothesis, Its Limitations, and Implications for Health and Disease." *Alternative Medicine Review*, August 2003.

[57] Cristea V. et al. "Lyme Disease with Magnesium Deficiency." *Magnesium Research* 16, no. 4 (Dec 2003): 287-9.

[58] Ibid.

[59] http://www.lowdosenaltrexone.org/

[60] Complete instructions may be found on Perque's website: http://www.perque.com/pdfs/Pt_Ascorbate_Flush_FINAL.pdf

[61] Darbinyan, V. et al. "Clinical Trial of Rhodiola Rosea L. Extract in the Treatment of Mild to Moderate Depression." *Nord J Psychiatry* 61, no. 5 (2007): 343-8.

[62] Ware, James R., trans. Alchemy, Medicine and Religion in the China of A.D. 320: The Nei Pien of Ko Hung. New York: Dover, 1966. 258.

[63] Cohen, Peta. "Interview with Dr. Cohen Concerning Biofilms and Enzyme Therapies." *PPTU Forum*. n.d. http://pptu.lefora.com/2011/01/17/interview-with-dr-cohen-concerning-biofilms-and-en/ (accessed March 2012).

[64] Duke, 2000, 216.

[65] Konlee, 1996.

[66] Mowrey, 1991.

[67] Duffell, Erika. "Curative Power of Fever." **The Lancet** 358, no. 9289 (2001): 1276-77.

[68] Barnes, 1976.

[69] De Maio, A. "Heat Shock Proteins: Facts, Thoughts, and Dreams." *Shock 11*, no. 1 (1999): 1-12; Shah, S. K. et al. "An Evidence-Based Review of a Lentinula Edodes Mushroom Extract as Complementary Therapy in the Surgical Oncology Patient." *Journal of Parenteral and Enteral Nutrition* 3 3 (2011).

[70] Santoro, M. G. "Heat Shock Factors and the Control of the Stress Response." Biochemical Pharmacology 59, no. 1 (2000): 55-63.

[71] Porcella, Stephen, et al. "Borrelia Burgdorferi and Treponema Pallidum: a Comparison of Functional Genomics, Environmental Adaptations, and Pathogenic Mechanisms." *Journal of Clinical Investigation* 107, no. 6 (March 2001): 651-56.

[72] Hydrotherapy is thoroughly covered in Boyle, 1988. If Amazon is too expensive, see http://www.eclecticherb.com/emp/ordering.html.

[73] See Thrash and Thrash for more on home heat therapies.

[74] Epsom Salt Industry Council. "Health Benefits of Epsom Salt Baths." http://www.care2.com/greenliving/health-benefits-of-epsom-salt-baths.html#ixzz1m7rLUD7C (accessed January 2012).

[75] Sven-Åke Bood. "Bending and Mending the Neurosignature: Frameworks of Influence by Floatation-REST." Karlstad University, 2007.

[76] Porcella, Stephen, et al. "Borrelia Burgdorferi and Treponema Pallidum: a Comparison of Functional Genomics, Environmental Adaptations, and Pathogenic Mechanisms."

*Journal of Clinical Investigation* 107, no. 6 (March 2001): 651-56.

[77] http://www.majidali.com/oxygen,_neuropathy,_and_healing.htm

[78] Ali, Majid. "Oxygen, Lyme Disease, and Fibromyalgia." http://majidalimd.wordpress.com. September 9, 2010. http://majidalimd.wordpress.com/2010/09/08/oxygen-lyme-disease-and-fibromyalgia/ (accessed November 23, 2010).

[79] Saul Pressman, email April 24, 2001. Used by permission.

[80] Warburg, Otto. "Preface to the Second Edition of the Lindau Lecture. The Prime Cause and Prevention of Cancer." Translated by Dean, National Cancer Institute, Bethesda, MD. Burk. Wurzburg: Konrad Triltsch, 1967. See also http://www.nobel.se/medicine/laureates/1931/press.html.

[81] Sweet, F., et al. "Ozone Selectively Inhibits Growth of Human Cancer Cells." *Science:* (72), p. 931 (1990).

[82] Much of this information is from Dr. Saul Pressman.

[83] Schunemann, H. J., et al. "Pulmonary Function Is a Long-term Predictor of Mortality in the General Population: 29-Year Follow-up of the Buffalo Health Study." *Chest* 118 (2000): 656-64.

[84] The complete Framingham study may be found at the National Institute of Health's Database: http://www.ncbi.nlm.nih.gov/PubMed/.

[85] Fried, 1999.

[86] von Ardenne, Manfred. *Oxygen Multistep Therapy: Physiological and Technical Foundations.* New York: Thieme New York, 1987.

[87] Cohen, 1997.

[88] Ibid., 178.

[89] Saraswati, 1978.

[90] Brown, Richard P., and Patricia L. Gerbarg. "Sudarshan Kriya Yogic Breathing in the Treatment of Stress, Anxiety, and Depression: Part I-Neurophysiologic Model." *J.Alternative and Complementary Medicine* 11, no. 1 (2005): 189-201.

[91] Ibid.

[92] http://www.himalayaninstitute.org/yoga-international-magazine/pranayama-articles/bhastrika-the-bellows-breath/

[93] Berendt, 1991,131.

[94] http://www.himalayaninstitute.org/yoga-international-magazine/pranayama-articles/

kapalabhati-the-skull-shining-breath/

[95] Cohen, 38-39.

[96] Olson, 159.

[97] Demos, 28–33.

[98] Le Scouamec, Rene-Pierre, et al. "Use of Binaural Beat Tapes for Treatment of Anxiety: A Pilot Study of Tape Preference and Outcomes." *Alternative Therapies in Health and Medicine* 7, no. 1 (2001).

[99] Demos, 201–7.

[100] Sojourner, 162.

[101] Gawain, 22-3.

[102] Gerard, 85-6.

# Index

51688222R00154

Made in the USA
Charleston, SC
31 January 2016